Controversies in Caring for Women with Epilepsy

Mona Sazgar • Cynthia L. Harden
Editors

Controversies in Caring for Women with Epilepsy

Sorting Through the Evidence

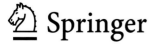 Springer

Editors
Mona Sazgar, M.D.
Clinical Professor
Department of Neurology
University of California, Irvine
Irvine, CA, USA

Cynthia L. Harden, M.D.
System Director of Epilepsy Services
Mount Sinai Health System
Mount Sinai Beth Israel Phillips
Ambulatory Care Center
New York, NY, USA

ISBN 978-3-319-29168-0   ISBN 978-3-319-29170-3   (eBook)
DOI 10.1007/978-3-319-29170-3

Library of Congress Control Number: 2016935404

Printed on acid-free paper

This Springer imprint is published by Springer Nature
The registered company is Springer International Publishing AG Switzerland

Foreword

"Example isn't another way to teach, it is the only way to teach."—Albert Einstein

Research on issues relating to women with epilepsy has expanded tremendously in the last two decades. Knowledge gained from the research has led to guidelines in the care of women with epilepsy. Major general neurology and epilepsy conferences consistently highlight topics regarding women with epilepsy. Yet, the care of each woman with epilepsy often requires more than knowledge and data. Clinical judgment that is evidence-supported is required to enable the selection and development of therapeutic strategies that may be suitable for each woman with epilepsy. The science of medicine based on data is often imperfect and insufficient to command a single therapeutic approach to a clinical scenario. This is where the art of medicine should come in—where the eye of the mind could critically appreciate the distinction and the overlap between therapeutic options that are reasonably viable for a specific clinical situation.

In this book, Dr. Sazgar and Dr. Harden have skillfully identified clinical scenarios that specially challenge clinicians to use scientific evidence to justify their recommendations for each scenario. The examples of contrasting options in the management of each clinical scenario underscore the complexities and vagaries in caring for women with epilepsy. The examples enhance learning of issues in women with epilepsy in a nuanced but more comprehensive manner, which will also help care providers in counseling women about their options for managing their epilepsy and related conditions.

Elson L. So, M.D.
President, American Epilepsy Society, 2014.

Preface

As epileptologists, each day Mona and I answer questions from women with epilepsy: "Will this medicine harm my baby?" "Will I be able to drive if I change medications?" "Will the seizures come back?" For each woman the stakes are high. As much as we wish for a single correct answer, the truth is that there exist multiple appropriate treatment approaches. We have created this book to explore expert guidance for office scenarios that are common, yet challenging. Since variation does exist even among experts, we are providing two expert approaches to the same vignette. It is our intent that this will be even more helpful than a single expert offering and will provide a well-rounded exploration of a specific medical situation in which a woman with epilepsy is seeking guidance. The reader can think about what considerations and decision pathways they take from each review. For example, management of a woman of reproductive age with juvenile myoclonic epilepsy is always at the top of the list of clinical conundrums. We have spun this scenario in many directions for our authors' input; for example, (1) the JME patient is stable taking valproate but has never tried any other antiseizure drugs, (2) the JME patient has failed all other antiseizure medications and is stable on valproate, and (3) the JME patient discovers that she is pregnant (9 weeks) and is stable on valproate.

Over the course of editing, Mona and I had the distinct pleasure of being a "fly on the wall" during the imaginary office visit. We have gained entrance onto the personal and warm conversations that the expert would have with the patient and family. Further, we are provided with the knowledge-based underpinnings for these discussions, and that is where it gets really interesting. All of the authors had strategies, algorithms, and supportive data for their decisions. The surprise is that many authors reached the same or similar conclusions based on differing sets of scientific evidence.

We are grateful to our contributors to agreeing to this format. Within a chapter, the specific review is not attributed to a specific author, but each author gets credit for the chapter. Therefore, we have implicitly gotten the authors to agree to disagree, should their responses differ. I will not reveal more about the "Controversies" in this preface, and I am sure that you will enjoy these short and to-the-point chapters and learn from them. I hope you will feel transported like I did to be actually in the room with an esteemed expert (although you won't know which one of the two it is!).

My respect and admiration for my contributing colleagues grows even greater now because I see how they work in an era in which obstacles to the therapeutic relationship are increasingly introduced. I would score all of the contributors at 100 % on any feedback scale for their impervious compassion and wisdom. Please allow this book to enrich your knowledge and enlarge your world a bit as you navigate through the "Controversies."

New York, NY   Cynthia L. Harden, M.D.

Contents

Part I Adolescence

1 **New Onset Primary Generalized Epilepsy in Adolescence** 3
   Daniel W. Shrey and Line Sveberg

2 **New Onset Partial Epilepsy in Adolescence** 11
   Patty McGoldrick, Steven M. Wolf, and Mary L. Zupanc

3 **Catamenial Epilepsy in Adolescence** 21
   Erika S. Pietzsch and Scott J. Stevens

4 **Contraception Choice in Adolescence** 29
   Barry E. Gidal, Mindl M. Messinger, and Katherine Noe

Part II Pre-Conception Counseling

5 **Folic Acid Supplementation** 39
   Kaarkuzhali Babu Krishnamurthy and George Lee Morris III

6 **Risk of Seizure During Pregnancy** 45
   Ajith Cherian, John C. DeToledo, Sahawat Tantikittichaikul,
   and Sanjeev V. Thomas

7 **Seizure Medications and Teratogenicity** 55
   David E. Friedman and Torbjörn Tomson

8 **Valproic Acid and Pregnancy: Failed Other Medications** 63
   Fábio A. Nascimento, Lara V. Marcuse, and Danielle M. Andrade

9 **Valproic Acid and Pregnancy: Not Tried Other Medications** 73
   Nigar Dargah-zada, Cynthia L. Harden, and Anne Sabers

10 **Epilepsy Inheritance** 81
   Madeline Fields and Mona Sazgar

11 **Infertility and Menstrual Disorders: Seizure Medications
    vs. Seizures**.. 87
    Esther Bui and Cynthia L. Harden

12 **Ever Advise Against Pregnancy?**.. 99
    Mona Sazgar and Frank J.E. Vajda

Part III   Pregnancy/Breast Feeding

13 **New Onset Seizures During Pregnancy** 107
    Chellamani Harini and Lilit Mnatsakanyan

14 **Valproic Acid and Pregnancy**.. 115
    Jakob Christensen and Sean Tchanho Hwang

15 **Lamotrigine and Pregnancy**.. 125
    Jennifer L. Hopp and David G. Vossler

16 **What Is Your Advice to Pregnant Women with Epilepsy
    Regarding Breastfeeding?** 133
    Kimford J. Meador and Gyri Veiby

Part IV   Menopause

17 **Change in Seizure Pattern and Menopause**.. 141
    Elizabeth E. Gerard, Sheryl Haut, and Puja Patel

18 **Perimenopausal Symptoms in Women with Epilepsy** 153
    Nitin K. Sethi and Mark S. Yerby

19 **Bone Health in Women with Epilepsy**... 159
    Pamela Crawford and Enrique A. Serrano

Index.. 169

Contributors

Danielle M. Andrade, M.D., M.Sc. Medical Director, Epilepsy Program, Krembil Neuroscience, Director of Epilepsy Genetics Research Program, Director, Epilepsy Transition Program, Associate Professor, Neurology, University of Toronto, Toronto, ON, Canada

Esther Bui, M.D., F.R.C.P.C. Neurology Comprehensive Epilepsy Program, Toronto Western Hospital, University of Toronto, Toronto, ON, Canada

Ajith Cherian, M.D., D.M. post doctoral fellow (Epilepsy) Department of Neurology, Sree Chitra Institute of Medical Sciences and Technology, Trivandrum, Kerala, India

Jakob Christensen, Ph.D., M.D. Department of Neurology, Aarhus University Hospital, Aarhus, Denmark

Pamela Crawford, M.B. Ch.B., M.D., F.R.C.P. Retired Consultant Neurologist, Department of Neurosciences, York Hospital, York, UK

Nigar Dargah-zada, M.D. Department of Neurology, Mount Sinai Beth Israel, New York, NY, USA

John C. DeToledo, M.D. Department of Neurology, Texas Tech University Health Sciences Center School of Medicine, Lubbock, TX, USA

Madeline Fields, M.D. Department of Neurology, The Mount Sinai Hospital, New York, NY, USA

David E. Friedman, M.D. Department of Neuroscience, Winthrop Comprehensive Epilepsy Center, Winthrop University Hospital, Mineola, NY, USA

Associate Clinical Professor of Neurology, SUNY Stony Brook School of Medicine, Mineola, NY, USA

Elizabeth E. Gerard, M.D. Department of Neurology, Feinberg School of Medicine, Chicago, IL, USA

Barry E. Gidal, Pharm.D. University of Wisconsin School of Pharmacy, Madison, WI, USA

Chellamani Harini, M.D. Division of Neurophysiology, Boston Children's Hospital, Boston, MA, USA

Sheryl Haut, M.D. Department of Neurology, Montefiore Medical Center, Albert Einstein College of Medicine, Bronx, NY, USA

Jennifer L. Hopp, M.D. Department of Neurology, University of Maryland School of Medicine, Maryland Epilepsy Center, Baltimore, MD, USA

Sean Tchanho Hwang, M.D. Department of Neurology, North Shore University Hospital, Hofstra North Shore LIJ Comprehensive Epilepsy Care Center, Great Neck, NY, USA

Kaarkuzhali Babu Krishnamurthy, B.S.E.E., M.D. Director, Women's Health in Epilepsy, Co-chair, Ethics Advisory Committee, Department of Neurology, Beth Israel Deaconess Medical Center, Boston, MA, USA

Lara V. Marcuse, M.D. Department of Neurology, Mount Sinai, New York, NY, USA

Patty McGoldrick, N.P. Department of Pediatric Neurology, Mount Sinai Health systems, New York, NY, USA

Kimford J. Meador, M.D. Department of Neurology & Neurological Sciences, Stanford University, Palo Alto, CA, USA

Mindl M. Messinger, Pharm.D. Pharmacy Department, Texas Children's Hospital, Houston, TX, USA

Lilit Mnatsakanyan, M.D. Department of Neurology, University of California Irvine Medical Center, Orange, CA, USA

George Lee Morris III, M.D. Aurora Health Care, St. Luke's Medical Center, Milwaukee, WI, USA

Center for Urban Population Health, Milwaukee, WI, USA

Zilber School of Public Health, Milwaukee, WI, USA

UW School of Public Health and Medicine, UW-Madison, Madison, WI, USA

Marquette University, Milwaukee, WI, USA

Epilepsy Center, St. Luke's Medical Center, Milwaukee, WI, USA

Fábio A. Nascimento, M.D. Division of Neurology, Toronto Western Hospital, University of Toronto, Toronto, ON, Canada

Katherine Noe, M.D., Ph.D. Department of Neurology, Mayo Clinic Arizona, Phoenix, AZ, USA

Puja Patel, M.D. Department of Neurology, Montefiore Medical Center, Albert Einstein College of Medicine, Bronx, NY, USA

Erika S. Pietzsch, M.D. Department of Neurology, Irvine, CA, USA

Anne Sabers, M.D., D.M.Sc. Department of Neurology, Rigshospitalet, Copenhagen, Denmark

Enrique A. Serrano, M.D. Department of Neurology, Comprehensive Epilepsy Center, University of Miami, Miller School of Medicine, Miami, FL, USA

Nitin K. Sethi, M.D., M.B.B.S., F.A.A.N. Department of Neurology, New York-Presbyterian Hospital, Weill Cornell Medical Center, New York, NY, USA

Daniel W. Shrey, M.D. Division of Neurology, Children's Hospital of Orange County, Department of Pediatrics, University of California Irvine, Orange, CA, USA

Scott J. Stevens, M.D. Department of Neurology, Hofstra North Shore—LIJ School of Medicine, Cushing Neuroscience Institute, Great Neck, NY, USA

Line Sveberg, M.D., Ph.D. Department of Neurology, Oslo University Hospital, Oslo, Norway

Sahawat Tantikittichaikul, M.D. Department of Neurology, Texas Tech University Health Sciences Center School of Medicine, Lubbock, TX, USA

Sanjeev V. Thomas, M.D., D.M. Department of Neurology, Sree Chitra Institute of Medical Sciences and Technology, Trivandrum, Kerala, India

Torbjörn Tomson, M.D., Ph.D. Department of Neurology, Karolinska University Hospital, Stockholm, Sweden

Frank J.E. Vajda, MB, BS, MD, FRCP, FRACP Department of Medicine and Neuroscience, Royal Melbourne Hospital, Melbourne, VIC, Australia

Gyri Veiby, M.D., Ph.D. Department of Neurology, Haukeland University Hospital, Bergen, Norway

David G. Vossler, M.D., F.A.A.N. Valley Medical Center, Neuroscience Institute, University of Washington, Renton, WA, USA

Steven M. Wolf, M.D. Department of Pediatric Neurology, Mount Sinai Health systems, New York, NY, USA

Mark S. Yerby, M.D., M.P.H. North Pacific Epilepsy Research, Bend, OR, USA

Mary L. Zupanc, M.D. Department of Pediatric Neurology, CHOC Children's Hospital/University of California, Irvine, Orange, CA, USA

Part I
Adolescence

Chapter 1
New Onset Primary Generalized Epilepsy in Adolescence

Daniel W. Shrey and Line Sveberg

Case Scenario

A 15-year-old girl has been having difficulties with clumsiness and dropping objects. These episodes have started in the past year, and are increasing in frequency and intensity. They occur more commonly in the early hours of the morning. Last week after she dropped and broke her glass of orange juice following a sudden involuntary jerk of her hand, she finally decided it is time to see her doctor who subsequently referred her to you for neurology consult. On further questioning, she does have a cousin with epilepsy and when in elementary school was noted by teachers to have episodes of daydreaming. She is a good student receiving As and Bs in most of her subjects in high school. Her neurologic exam is normal. Her EEG shows generalized 4 Hz spike-and-wave discharges as well as a few fragments of spikes in the frontotemporal areas bilaterally. What is your decision pathway in terms of diagnostic and treatment approaches for her?

D.W. Shrey, M.D.
Division of Neurology, Children's Hospital of Orange County,
Department of Pediatrics, University of California Irvine,
1201 W La Veta Ave, Orange, CA 92868, USA

L. Sveberg, M.D., Ph.D.
Department of Neurology, Oslo University Hospital,
Sognsvannsveien 20, 0372 Oslo, Norway
e-mail: line.sveberg@ous-hf.no

Commentator: M. Sazgar, M.D. (✉)
University of California, Irvine Medical Center,
101 The City Drive South, Pavilion I, Bldg. 30, Suite 123, Orange, CA 92868, USA
email: msazgar@uci.edu

© Springer International Publishing Switzerland 2016
M. Sazgar, C.L. Harden (eds.), *Controversies in Caring for Women with Epilepsy*, DOI 10.1007/978-3-319-29170-3_1

AUTHOR #1'S RESPONSE

Evaluation of an adolescent girl with suspected seizures and epileptic EEG involves a multitude of diagnostic and treatment considerations. Being on the cusp of adulthood, she can be perceived as standing at a crossroad from where, in the years immediately ahead, she will make decisions that will have a profound impact on her life in terms of both future profession(s) and relationship(s). A diagnosis and subsequent treatment of epilepsy will be therefore of particular importance. The ultimate aim is that these critical years will not be blemished by unpredicted seizures or troublesome side effects of medications. Thus, a certainty of diagnosis and a well-reflected treatment choice are critical.

In the first consultation with the patient and her parents, the best description of her possible seizures must be clearly established. The parents should be asked non-leading questions regarding how the teachers reported her tendency to daydream as a child. Her current symptoms of clumsiness could surely be classified as being among the well-known behavior of a careless teenager, but the escalation of these symptoms and the additional information of an epileptic EEG prompt further investigation into this phenomenon. The parents should be further asked about what happens when she drops objects or is visibly clumsy; could these episodes be characterized as sudden, brief, lightening-like muscle jerks?

Finally, in the search for evidence of different types of epileptic seizures, consideration should be given to signs of seizures that have not yet been perceived as such or not perceived at all. Signs of tongue or lip bites in the morning could be evidence of nightly generalized tonic-clonic seizures (GTCS). In this summary, however, no indications of GTCS are provided. With the result of the EEG in hand and a characteristic description, retrospective evaluation might suggest that both the daydreaming episodes and the clumsiness incident are probably epileptic events, with absences in childhood and myoclonias in adolescence being the most probable seizure semiology in this teenage girl. Her myoclonus on awakening that is associated with typical generalized epileptiform EEG, together with her age and normal intelligence, fulfills the class I diagnostic criteria for juvenile myoclonus epilepsy (JME) [1]. In many JME patients, absence seizures may be the first seizure type. In this patient, who has generalized epileptic activity on EEG, it might be assumed that her propensity for childhood daydreaming represented absences.

In an affluent society, cerebral MRI is usually warranted in newly diagnosed epilepsy cases; it is expected that doctors will do everything possible to find the cause of unexpected illness in a child. In this patient, however, who is obtaining high grades and has a normal neurological status, with predominantly generalized discharges on the EEG, the chances of finding relevant pathology are rather low.

Although she has not had any GTCS, the seizure semiology and the EEG results consistent with a diagnosis of JME indicate that there should be an evaluation of antiepileptic drug (AED) treatment.

Valproate is acknowledged as the most effective drug in the treatment of JME. However, due to its side effects, the relevant guidelines warn against its use in young women. Weight gain and excessive hair growth are not popular side effects, particularly in this age group, but it is the increased potential for teratogenic and cognitive effects on the child that has strengthened the basis for this advice [2, 3]. It has been proposed that lower doses of valproate may not be associated with this increased risk, but, nevertheless, in general, valproate is not recommended unless other treatments are not tolerated or are found to be ineffective.

An alternative treatment for this generalized epilepsy is lamotrigine (LTG). LTG is generally well-tolerated if slowly titrated, but pregnancy and the use of contraception should also be discussed as both pregnancy and the use of oral contraceptives are known to enhance the metabolism of LTG and decrease its serum levels [4]. LTG may also have less effect on myoclonus which is her current symptom.

Levetiracetam (LEV) is another potential alternative AED for this patient. LEV treatment may increase psycholability or cause behavioral side effects that are not easily monitored in an adolescent. Not having had any of these problems prior to treatment, it might be suggested that this patient may be less prone to develop these kinds of side effects.

Topiramate and zonisamide are other possible treatments for JME. However, the side effects of these medications include weight loss and cognitive effects, and also a potential for teratogenicity, although this has been the subject of fewer investigations.

The patient is a young girl, unaccustomed to daily medication, and after hearing of possible side effects, she or her parents may hesitate to start on treatment with an AED, and may advocate that her current seizures, the myoclonias, are tolerable. This perspective may be reinforced by the fact that she is also a good student and with no indication of neuropsychological implications due to seizures. This point of view should be acknowledged and discussed. However, her myoclonias have been noted to be increasing, and with the EEG exhibiting generalized epileptic discharges, a future escalation in her seizure frequency or severity is highly probable. A generalized seizure could cause injuries or worse complications, depending on the situation. A GTCS would also postpone her chances of obtaining a driver's license and could create a significant social impact during a very vulnerable life-period. The teenage years also harbor the probability of increased exposure to typical seizure-triggers, such as sleep deprivation and binge drinking.

My recommendation would therefore be AED treatment. The choice between LTG and LEV is not as clear-cut, but LEV could be chosen here because the effect of LTG on myoclonias is less efficient. However, the final choice should only be made after a good discursive consultation, including the aspects mentioned above, and taking into account the attitude of the patient and also the parents' values and comments.

In summary, an adolescent girl with probable absences in childhood, morning myoclonias, and generalized seizure activity on EEG is diagnosed as suffering from JME. Treatment options should be carefully discussed because side effects and efficacies have many implications for her future quality of life.

AUTHOR #2'S RESPONSE

In this case, the patient's clinical history is most consistent with a diagnosis of primary generalized epilepsy. Elements of the clinical history that are supportive of primary generalized epilepsy include onset of symptoms during childhood/adolescence, family history of epilepsy, and normal cognitive function as well as a normal neurological exam. Her history of staring spells as a child raises concern for prior absence seizures and when coupled with her recent development of progressively worsening morning myoclonic jerks, is suggestive of a diagnosis of juvenile myoclonic epilepsy, or JME. A significant portion of patients diagnosed with JME also carry other seizure types, most commonly generalized tonic-clonic and, less frequently, absence seizures. The electrographic findings of generalized 4 Hz spike-and-slow-wave activity with fragmented bilateral frontotemporal spikes are also supportive of this diagnosis [5].

With respect to further diagnostic testing, many practitioners would consider confirming the diagnosis of JME by performing a long-term video EEG study that includes photic stimulation and hyperventilation. Ideally, such a study would capture and characterize her myoclonic jerks, query for subtle absence seizures, and also determine if she is among the almost 50 % of patients with JME who develop epileptiform discharges and/or myoclonic seizures during photic stimulation. This information would be beneficial when counselling her regarding lifestyle modifications that can minimize the chances of further seizures occurring. Genetic testing should be discussed, as she has a family history of epilepsy and JME has been shown to have a strong genetic component with multifactorial and complex inheritance patterns.

Regarding an approach to therapy, many factors should be considered. Typical first-line antiseizure medications used to treat JME include valproate, lamotrigine, and levetiracetam. Other agents, such as topiramate and zonisamide, show promise mostly as adjunctive agents.

Valproate is considered by many to be one of the most effective medications used to treat JME. It was shown by one study to effectively treat absence, myoclonic, and GTC seizures in 86 % of patients with JME [6]. Additionally, it has the added benefit of rapid titration to goal dosing and the ability to load intravenously in emergent situations. Drawbacks to valproate include its metabolic interactions with other medications as well as increased risk of liver failure, pancreatitis, and thrombocytopenia. In adolescent females, significant consideration should be given before starting valproate, as it is a known teratogen, often leads to weight gain, and also has been shown to increase the risk of polycystic ovaries and lead to hyperandrogenism in some women [7]. Additionally, offspring of women who use valproate during pregnancy are at increased risk of having significant neurodevelopmental delay [8]. It has also been reported to cause hair loss. Often times, these side effects prompt neurologists and patients to prefer other antiseizure medications when the first monotherapy agent is selected in a young woman with JME.

Lamotrigine is another viable option. It has considerably lower teratogenicity compared to valproate and has proven efficacy in treating generalized seizures, however, it was shown to be inferior to valproate in treating idiopathic generalized epilepsy [9]. One considerable drawback to lamotrigine therapy is the length of time from onset of treatment until the goal dose is reached. Most providers will increase the medication over 2–3 months in order to minimize the risks of Stevens Johnson Syndrome. In this patient's case, where she has not yet had any GTCS, there is less urgency than is present when a JME patient has already experienced several GTCS prior to starting their first antiseizure medication. Additionally, a significant minority of patients with JME may have worsening of their myoclonus while taking lamotrigine.

Levetiracetam should also be considered, as it has known efficacy in treating myoclonus, is effective at treating generalized seizures, has less medication and liver interactions than the other two medications, and can be quickly increased to goal dosing. Like valproate, it can be loaded intravenously as well. Levetiracetam also has little to no known effects on the endocrine system [8]. Additionally, pregnancy registry data suggests a low teratogenic risk when taken while pregnant. One drawback to using levetiracetam in children is that it has been shown to cause increased irritability and behavioral disturbances in a minority of patients.

The treatment of refractory JME involves consideration for many other antiseizure medications, including topiramate and zonisamide. Rational polytherapy usually plays a strong initial role. Consideration should be given to usage of the modified Atkins or ketogenic diet for more refractory cases.

After establishing a diagnosis of JME, I would first counsel this patient regarding lifestyle modifications that have been shown to minimize the risk of seizures and improve quality of life in patients with JME. I would advise her to avoid drinking alcohol, to establish excellent sleep hygiene and minimize sleep deprivation, and also to avoid photic stimulation if she is found to be photosensitive. I would also strongly recommend strict antiseizure medication compliance, as the majority of patients with JME can remain seizure free on monotherapy if their medication is taken properly and they avoid precipitating circumstances.

For initial antiseizure medication monotherapy, my treatment of choice would most likely be levetiracetam in this patient. Myoclonic seizures are her predominant seizure type at this time, and levetiracetam has proven efficacy with myoclonic seizures as well as generalized seizures. Should she prove to be refractory to levetiracetam, I would try lamotrigine next, given its superior side-effect profile to valproate, especially in young women. If she fails lamotrigine as well, I would consider adding low-dose valproate as an adjunctive therapy while closely monitoring lamotrigine levels due to the known enzymatic interactions between the two drugs. Low-dose valproate is associated with lower risk of poor neurodevelopmental outcome compared to higher dosages [8]. I would also counsel her appropriately regarding the reproductive side effects of her medication(s).

Reviewer's Comments

This case scenario is depicting the challenges of counselling adolescent female and her family regarding a new diagnosis of epilepsy and the need to make changes in lifestyle and assume responsibility of taking daily seizure medication. Author #1 and Author #2 both agree with diagnosis of JME in this 15-year-old young lady. Both authors agree in starting her on anticonvulsant therapy and both suggest levetiracetam as the first choice due to patient's prominent myoclonic seizures. Both practitioners suggest lamotrigine as the second choice of therapy due to less favorable side effect profile of valproic acid in young women with epilepsy. Topiramate and zonisamide are lower on their list due to potential cognitive side effects.

Both authors point out the importance of extensive counselling of the patient and her family regarding the implications of epilepsy diagnosis and treatment or lack of treatment. The potential restriction of driving and social impact of seizure recurrence, specially a tonic-clonic seizure, is discussed by these authors. They both advise the patient to avoid sleep deprivation and excessive alcoholic beverage consumption. Second author adds the caution against photic triggers in case of photosensitive epilepsy.

Levetiracetam in the United States is approved by Food and Drug Administration (FDA) as adjunctive therapy for use in myoclonic seizures in patients 12 years and older with JME and for idiopathic primary generalized epilepsy in patients 6 years and older. The European Medical Agency (EMA) does not give levetiracetam an indication for monotherapy. However, it is frequently used as monotherapy in women of childbearing age for its superior risk benefit ratio in these women. Lamotrigine is FDA approved for adjunctive therapy in idiopathic primary generalized epilepsy in patients 2 years and older. Valproate has monotherapy indication for absence seizures. The only medication with approved FDA indication for monotherapy in primary generalized epilepsy in the United States is topiramate.

The most recent expert recommendation from a joint Task Force of ILAE-commission on European Affairs and European Academy of Neurology [10] discourages using valproate as first-line therapy in girls and women of childbearing age with newly diagnosed epilepsy. Despite being considered the most effective therapy for JME, its use should be limited due to potential teratogenic and neurocognitive side effects on the fetus and multiple long-term side effects on young women including but not limited to polycystic ovarian syndrome, hyperandrogenism, weight gain, liver, and pancreatic toxicity.

In brief, the comments of our two contributors and review of the available data suggest a general agreement in management of the presented case vignette in this chapter.

Suggested Management

1. Counsel the patient and family regarding the diagnosis of JME, potential risks and benefits of starting medication and lifestyle implications.

2. Patient to avoid sleep deprivation, excessive EtOH use, and in case of light-sensitive epilepsy, exposure to flashing light.
3. Consider levetiracetam for cases with prominent myoclonic component.
4. Consider lamotrigine if sufficient time allows for slow titration.
5. Valproic acid, topiramate, and zonisamide use will need significant risk benefit consideration and mostly use if other treatment options fail.

References

1. Penry JK, Dean JC, Riela AR. Juvenile myoclonic epilepsy: long-term response to therapy. Epilepsia. 1989;30 Suppl 4:S19–23. discussion S24–S27.
2. Harden CL, Pennel PB. Neuroendocrine considerations in the treatment of men and women with epilepsy. Lancet Neurol. 2013;12(1):72–83.
3. Meador KJ, Baker GA, et al. Cognitive function at 3 years of age after fetal exposure to anti-epileptic drugs. N Engl J Med. 2009;360(16):1597–605.
4. Marson AG, et al. The SANAD study of effectiveness of valproate, lamotrigine, or topiramate for generalized and unclassifiable epilepsy: an unblended randomized controlled trial. Lancet. 2007;369(9566):1016–26.
5. Kasteleijn-Nolst Trenité DG, Semitz B, Janz D, Delgado-Escuita AV, Thomas P, Hirsch E, et al. Consensus on diagnosis and management of JME: from founder's observations to current trends. Epilepsy Behav. 2013;28:S87–90.
6. Tomson T, Marson A, Boon P, Canevini MP, Covanis A, Gaily E, et al. Valproate in the treatment of epilepsy in women and girls. Pre-publication summary of recommendations from a joint Task Force of ILAE-commission on European Affairs and European Academy of Neurology (EAN). Eur Acad Neurol. 2015; 10 March.
7. Bromley R, Weston J, Adab N, Greenhalgh J, Sanniti A, McKay AJ, et al. Treatment for epilepsy in pregnancy: neurodevelopment outcomes in the child. Cochrane Database Syst Rev. 2014;10:CD010236. doi:10.1002/14651858.CD010236.pub2.
8. Ohman I, Luef G, Tomson T. Effects of pregnancy and contraception on lamotrigine disposition: new insights through analysis of lamotrigine metabolites. Seizure. 2008;17(2):199–202.
9. Panayiotopoulos CP, Obeid T, Tahan AR. Juvenile myoclonic epilepsy: a 5-year prospective study. Epilepsia. 1994;35(2):285–96.
10. Tomson T, Marson A, Boon P, Canevini MP, Covanis A, Gaily E, et al. Valproate in the treatment of epilepsy in girls and women of childbearing potential. Epilepsia. 2015;56:1006–19.

Chapter 2
New Onset Partial Epilepsy in Adolescence

Patty McGoldrick, Steven M. Wolf, and Mary L. Zupanc

Case Scenario

An 18-year-old right-handed neurologically normal woman has new onset focal epilepsy, presenting with a secondary generalized tonic-clonic seizure after a year-long history of episodes of déjà vu associated with mild confusion lasting 1–2 min. She has a normal MRI, no risk factors for epilepsy, and an EEG that shows right temporal spikes. What is your decision pathway in terms of diagnostic and treatment approaches for her?

P. McGoldrick, N.P. • S.M. Wolf, M.D.
Department of Pediatric Neurology, Mount Sinai Health systems,
10 Union Square East, Suite 5G, New York, NY 10003, USA
e-mail: pmcgoldr@chpnet.org; swolf@chpnet.org

M.L. Zupanc, M.D.
Department of Pediatric Neurology, CHOC Children's Hospital/University of California, Irvine, 1201 W. La Veta Ave, Orange, CA 92868, USA
e-mail: mzupanc@choc.org

Commentator: C.L. Harden, M.D. (✉)
Mount Sinai Health System, Mount Sinai Beth Israel Phillips Ambulatory Care Center,
10 Union Square East, Suite 5D, New York, NY10003, USA
e-mail: charden@chpnet.org

AUTHOR #1'S RESPONSE

Evaluation

Step One

Review the MRI with a radiologist with experience in epilepsy as well as with an epileptologist.

Step Two

An overnight EEG should be ordered, either ambulatory or inpatient, to determine the extent of epileptiform abnormalities in sleep and awake and determine risk of future seizures.

Step Three

Classify the seizures as best as you can! Get a good description of her event including the feelings or auras that the patient experienced before the clinical seizure, the actual presentation, how long it lasted, and how long until it generalized. This will aid in determining the area of seizure onset and help to decide future treatment options including epileptic surgery if the seizures do not respond to treatment with medications.

Step Four: Treatment Options

1. Wait: Watch to see if more events occur. If this was an isolated incident and the patient had not reported auras, it would be reasonable to wait and see if she had another seizure over the next 6–12 months before initiating treatment.
2. Treat: In this case the patient has auras and an abnormal EEG. There is a risk of recurrent seizures and it is prudent to initiate treatment with medication. When choosing medications for treatment of seizures, the provider must first determine whether the medication is appropriate for the treatment of focal seizures.

Things to Consider

It is important to get to know your patient—where is she in her life? Starting college, moving out, starting a job, starting a family? The provider needs to consider certain things:

1. Body image issues: Will the medication cause weight loss or weight gain? In adolescent girls, most providers will want to avoid medications that increase appetite and can cause weight gain. However, if the patient is underweight, medications that decrease appetite should be avoided. Weight should be monitored during treatment.

2. Childbearing potential: Will any of the medications cause infertility or are they teratogenic? Pregnancy registries are our best sources of information regarding outcomes. Women with epilepsy are known to be less fertile than other women [1] but there is no evidence to suggest that certain anti-epileptic drugs (AEDs) cause a decrease in fertility. Some medications are teratogenic and should be avoided in pregnancy and in women of childbearing potential, because of a risk of impaired fine motor skills and social skills and major congenital malformations in their offspring [2].

3. Drug-to-drug interactions: It is important to consider the interaction of the anti-seizure medication with medications used for other medical conditions. In this case, the patient has no medical history, but if she had a chronic illness — asthma, cardiac disease, or diabetes, interactions would have to be checked.

4. Contraception: Some contraceptives decrease the efficacy of antiepileptic medications. Some AEDs decrease the efficacy of hormonal contraceptives and therefore alternate birth control options should be explored (see Table 2.1). Contraceptives are sometimes used in catamenial epilepsy to decrease frequency and length of menses, thereby decreasing seizures [3].

5. Neuropsychiatric side effects: Some medications can cause irritability and even psychosis, while others are mood stabilizing. Supplementation with vitamin B6 can prevent this side effect. Often, persons newly diagnosed with epilepsy become depressed and/or anxious. This should be closely monitored.

6. Monitoring: This includes the need for blood levels, CBC, chemistry, liver function tests, and chemistry (all of which are specific to the AED prescribed). The provider should also determine how often the EEG and a prolonged EEG should be repeated and whether or not the neuroimaging study should be repeated, perhaps using an epilepsy surgery protocol. Typically, this would be required if the seizures become intractable.

7. Supplements: All women should be supplemented with Calcium and vitamin D. Women of childbearing age should receive folic acid supplementation to reduce the risk for fetal birth defects.

8. Breast feeding: Recent studies show that antiepileptic medication is safe in breastfeeding [4].

9. Driving: In many states, providers are mandated to report persons with epilepsy to the Department of Motor Vehicles. Laws may restrict driving for a certain period of time after a seizure, although some states make allowances for breakthrough seizures that occur with medication changes.

10. Lifestyles: Alcohol, marijuana, adherence to regimen, late nights, school notification, and marriage notification. The patient in question is 18 years old. In some cultures, she is achieving independence by working. In others, she is in college; and in some she may be preparing for marriage. It is important to choose medications that will provide good seizure control even

Table 2.1 Medication in focal epilepsy

Generic name	Brand name	Mechanism of action	Teratogenicity	Interaction with hormonal contraceptives	Effect on weight	Comments
Carbamazepine	Carbatrol, tegretol	Blocks sodium channels	Neural tube defects	Decrease efficacy of OCP	Increased	Monitor blood levels – may lower sodium
Oxcarbazepine	Trileptal	Blocks sodium channels	Inadequate data	Decrease efficacy of OCP	Neutral (increased)	May lower sodium
Levetiracetam	Keppra	Inhibits sodium channels	Low rate of defects; no specific type	Weak enzyme inducer/ inhibitor	Neutral	Side effect of irritability
Valproic acid	Depakote	Increases GABA, may inhibit glutamate/NMDA	Neural tube defects and lowering of IQ	CYP450	Increased	Not with PCOS or DM – monitor blood levels – may decrease platelets and effect liver
Eslicarbazepine acetate	Aptiom	Inhibits sodium channels	No data	Reduces efficacy of oral contraceptives	Neutral	Monitor sodium
Topiramate	Topamax, Trokendi, Qudexy	Blocks voltage-dependent sodium channels; augments GABA, antagonizes glutamate receptors, and inhibits carbonic anhydrase	Cleft palate	None	Decreased	Can cause renal stones, glaucoma
Lacosamide	Vimpat	Enhances slow inactivation of voltage-sensitive sodium channels	Insufficient data	Prolongs PR interval	Neutral	Contraindicated with cardiac failure
Lamotrigine	Lamictal	Sodium channels	Cleft lip and palate	Decrease efficacy of OCP	Neutral	Risk of Stevens-Johnson sx

if she is using recreational drugs, like alcohol and marijuana and even when she is sleep-deprived. The provider needs to discuss the fact that alcohol, marijuana with a high THC content, and sleep deprivation lower the seizure threshold. She should be encouraged to abstain from the use of recreational drugs, get adequate sleep each night (no pulling all-nighters to study) and that the medication MUST be taken as prescribed and at approximately the same time every day. Patients are more compliant when medications are dosed once a day, so the use of extended release medications is encouraged. However, we have found that in some active adolescents, the extended release formulations still need to be taken twice a day. As for marriage, if this girl is about to enter into marriage, it is likely that the other family will require assurance that the epilepsy is not genetically mediated.

11. Menstrual concerns/Catamenial epilepsy refers to epilepsies in which seizures occur more frequently around menses and ovulation, occurring in about 35 % of women with epilepsy, independent of the type of seizure or its etiology [5]. The hypothesis is that cortical excitability varies with hormonal fluctuation in women with epilepsy [6].

12. Other tests: If this patient's seizures become intractable, treatment options include ketogenic diet, non-lesional resective surgery, vagal nerve stimulator, and responsive neurostimulation. Evaluation for surgery would necessitate a repeat MRI, video EEG, neuropsychological testing, functional MRI, and possibly a Wada.

In conclusion, in caring for this adolescent female with a history of auras and new onset of seizures, the decision pathway should include:

- A good evaluation
- Getting to know the patient
- Consideration of side effects when treating with medications
- Education
- Periodic reevaluation of treatment

AUTHOR #2'S RESPONSE

With respect to treatment options, there are several antiepileptic medications that could be considered. It is the responsibility of the physician to inform the patient that AED therapy is important and will, most likely, prevent further seizures. It is also the physician's responsibility to partner with the patient with respect to the available choices of AED therapy. The risks vs. benefits should be described in detail.

The possible AED options include:

1. Oxcarbazepine
2. Carbamazepine
3. Lamotrigine

4. Levetiracetam
5. Valproate

Levetiracetam is certainly an antiepileptic medication that should be considered. There are no known drug interactions. It does not affect the liver or bone marrow, being excreted primarily through the kidney. It rarely produces an allergic drug rash and does not affect neurocognitive functioning. Its primary side effects include behavioral disinhibition and psychiatric effects, including increased risk of suicidal thoughts. For an adolescent with a tendency for anxiety and/or depression, this might not be the best choice. With respect to reproductive health, the initial pregnancy registry data suggests a low risk for major congenital malformations.

Oxcarbazepine or carbamazepine could be considered for this young woman. These two antiepileptic medications are generally well tolerated at therapeutic dosages and equally effective in the treatment of partial epilepsy [7]. If high dosages are required, there may be cognitive side effects. In addition, weight gain can be seen with both of these medications. Oxcarbazepine does not produce the epoxide metabolite, which is felt to be responsible for the primary side effects of carbamazepine, including nausea, vomiting, diplopia, fatigue, and ataxia.

With respect to reproductive health, carbamazepine does carry a risk of major congenital anomalies, including neural tube defects and oral clefts. The teratogenic effects of oxcarbazepine are yet to be fully defined. If this adolescent chooses to go on oral contraceptives or use Depo-Provera, she should be informed that both carbamazepine and oxcarbazepine are P450 enzyme inducers, but carbamazepine is the more potent inducer. Oral contraceptives and Depo-Provera are metabolized by the P450 enzyme system. Therefore, if an oral contraceptive is chosen, it must contain relatively high-dose estrogen (50 micrograms). The Depo-provera injections need to be given more frequently than in someone who is not taking an enzyme-inducing drug [8, 9].

In summary, both carbamazepine and oxcarbazepine are effective in the treatment of partial epilepsy. However, oxcarbazepine is preferable, given its better safety profile (less risk of idiosyncratic reactions), lack of autoinduction, low protein binding, linear pharmacokinetics, and minimal drug interactions, contraceptives excluded [7, 8].

Lamotrigine is another antiepileptic medication to consider for this young woman. It is well tolerated, with few side effects. It does not change a patient's neurocognitive profile, is a mood stabilizer, and can function as an antidepressant. Most patients like the fact that lamotrigine does not affect their cognitive abilities and improves their mood. There are a few patients who become more anxious on lamotrigine, and some may experience sleep disturbance. If this patient has obsessive compulsive tendencies, lamotrigine might exacerbate them.

One drawback of lamotrigine is that it requires a slow titration in order to avoid the risk of a serious allergic rash. In an adult patient, this risk (such as Steven's

Johnson syndrome) is approximately 0.3 %. If a patient is having frequent seizures, the lamotrigine titration process may be too risky. However, some physicians will use a bridging medication, such as clonazepam, as the lamotrigine is titrated into the therapeutic range.

With respect to reproductive health, lamotrigine does not affect estradiol metabolism, but does affect the levonorgestrel metabolism. No breakthrough ovulation has been reported, but oral contraceptives alone as a form of birth control may be inadequate. One pregnancy registry has reported an increased risk of cleft palate/cleft lip as a teratogenic side effect of lamotrigine. However, this has not been confirmed in other pregnancy registries [8, 9].

Valproate should not be used as a first choice antiepileptic medication in a young woman in the reproductive age. There are several reasons for this, including:

1. Valproate has been reported to cause menstrual irregularities and anovulatory cycles; hormonal changes such as hyperandrogenism and increased testosterone; hyperinsulinism; and polycystic ovaries. With respect to polycystic ovary syndrome and its association with valproate, the epilepsy itself, hypothalamic dysfunction, and additional factors may be also be contributory [10].
2. Valproate has proven teratogenic effects, including an increased risk of neural tube defects [8, 9].
3. In the NEAD study, children who have been exposed to valproate in utero and who had developmental assessments at age three were found to have significant cognitive impairments compared to children who had fetal exposure to other antiepileptic medications [11].

Phenobarbital would be relatively contraindicated in this young woman, due to its cognitive side effects. Phenytoin would also be relatively contraindicated due to its many side effects (cognitive slowing, coarsening of the facial features, hirsutism, osteoporosis, and teratogenic effects), its pharmacokinetics, and its many drug interactions.

Lacosamide is FDA approved as initial monotherapy or conversion to monotherapy and as adjunctive therapy in partial epilepsy. Lacosamide use in this clinical setting is limited by the lack of evidence for teratogenic risk. This limits the ability to counsel and discuss regarding its use. It does not interact with oral contraceptives however.

The optimal choices for this young woman would include: oxcarbazepine, levetiracetam, or lamotrigine. The choice would depend on the concurrent medical and psychiatric history, as well as the woman's own preferences.

Finally, if this woman's epilepsy is not controlled despite two trials of antiepileptic medication, appropriately chosen, with levels pushed to the high therapeutic range, she should be evaluated for epilepsy surgery. Her seizures appear to emanate from the right temporal lobe, probably nondominant. If the presurgical evaluation confirms this, she would fall into a favorable group for epilepsy surgery.

Reviewer's Comments

These two responses are very different in their emphasis, but between them, the diagnostic, treatment and counseling approaches for the 18-year-old woman with new onset focal epilepsy are encompassed. The contribution by Author #1 begins with a stepwise approach to understanding the exact epilepsy diagnosis and etiology. This is followed by a comprehensive approach to understanding the individual patient and her specific concerns and risk factors for medication side effects, seizure recurrence, and reproductive vulnerability. They point out that the query, "where are you in your life right now?" in terms of school, working, driving, romantic involvements and activities with friends is key to guiding medication choices. Author #2 accepted the premise that this is a newly diagnosed epilepsy patient and focused on her exact medication choices. These were oxcarbazepine, levetiracetam or lamotrigine, with details regarding the benefits and drawbacks of each choice for this patient. Both responses incorporated the need to tailor the treatment choice to fit the clinical scenario as well as involving the patient in the medication choice. Both responses concluded with consideration of epilepsy surgery if the patient does not respond to medication treatment, specifically stated in Author #2's contribution, "if this woman's epilepsy is not controlled despite two trials of antiepileptic medication, appropriately chosen, with levels pushed to the high therapeutic range, she should be evaluated for epilepsy surgery." Consideration of an epilepsy surgery evaluation for appropriate patients is always on the "front-burner" for epilepsy doctors. However, recent data show that in the pediatric age group, obstacles to the timely consideration of epilepsy surgery are both systematic and random. For example, the decision to move forward with epilepsy surgery is linked to difficult-to-quantify considerations such as the patient and family's acceptance of the option, the strength of the therapeutic alliance with the healthcare team, and the family's ability to absorb a likely financial setback [12]. While epilepsy surgery may be a consideration as this patient is assessed on an ongoing basis, the chapters here provide an excellent overview of initial management of this young focal epilepsy patient.

Suggested Management

1. Once the diagnosis of focal epilepsy is established, lamotrigine, oxcarbazepine, and levetiracetam are reasonable treatment options.
2. Current lifestyle and lifestyle goals are important considerations in guiding pharmacologic and non-pharmacologic management.
3. Pregnancy risks must be addressed for young women.
4. Early identification of antiseizure drug-resistant patients who may be candidates for surgical cure is important to mitigate a life trajectory turned downward by seizures.

References

1. Morrell MJ, Giudice L, Flynn KL, Seale CG, Paulson AJ, Done S, et al. Predictors of ovulatory failure in women with epilepsy. Ann Neurol. 2002;52:704–11.
2. Campbell E, Kennedy F, Russell A, Smithson WH, Parsons L, Morrison PJ, et al. Malformation risks of antiepileptic drug monotherapies in pregnancy: updated results from the UK and Ireland Epilepsy and Pregnancy Registers. J Neurol Neurosurg Psychiatry. 2014;85:1029–34.
3. Najafi M, Sadeghi MM, Mehvari J, Zare M, Akbari M. Progesterone therapy in women with intractable catamenial epilepsy. Adv Biomed Res. 2013;2:8.
4. Veiby G, Engelsen BA, Gilhus NE. Early child development and exposure to antiepileptic drugs prenatally and through breastfeeding: a prospective cohort study on children of women with epilepsy. JAMA Neurol. 2013;70:1367–74.
5. El-Khayat HA, Soliman NA, Tomoum HY, Omram MA, El-Wakad AS, Shatla RH. Reproductive hormonal changes and catamenial pattern in adolescent females with epilepsy. Epilepsia. 2008;49:1619–26.
6. Badawy RA, Vogrin SJ, Lai A, Cook MJ. Are patterns of cortical hyperexcitability altered in catamenial epilepsy? Ann Neurol. 2013;74:743–57.
7. Mintzer S, Mattson RT. Should enzyme-inducing antiepileptic drugs be considered first-line agents? Epilepsia. 2009;50 Suppl 8:42–50.
8. Pennell PB. Chapter 45: Treatment of epilepsy during pregnancy. In: Wyllie E, Cascino G, Gidal B, Goodkin H, editors. Wyllie's treatment of epilepsy: principles and practice. 5th ed. Philadelphia: Lippincott, Williams and Wilkins; 2011. p. 557–68.
9. Pennell PB. Pregnancy, epilepsy and women's issues. Continuum. 2013;19(3):697–714.
10. Harden CL, Pennell PB. Neuroendocrine considerations in the treatment of men and women with epilepsy. Lancet Neurol. 2013;12:72–83.
11. Meador KJ, Baker GA, Browning N, Clayton-Smith J, Combs-Cantrell DT, Cohen M, et al. Cognitive function at 3 years of age after fetal exposure to antiepileptic drugs. N Engl J Med. 2009;360:1597–605.
12. Baca CB, Pieters HC, Iwaki TJ, Mathern GW, Vickrey BG. "A journey around the world": parent narratives of the journey to pediatric resective epilepsy surgery and beyond. Epilepsia. 2015;56:822–32.

Chapter 3
Catamenial Epilepsy in Adolescence

Erika S. Pietzsch and Scott J. Stevens

Case Scenario

A 16-year-old woman with focal epilepsy has premenstrual focal seizures with dyscognitive features which occur within 3 days of her menstrual onset and occurring approximately six times per year. She has regular menses and is not on birth control. What is your sequence in evaluating and treating this patient and in managing this young woman with premenstrual seizure exacerbations?

AUTHOR #1'S RESPONSE

This is a young 16-year-old woman of childbearing age and expected excitements and changes in her life. There are multiple prospects that have to be discussed with the patient.

E.S. Pietzsch, M.D.
Department of Neurology, 4442 Spectrum, Irvine, CA 92618, USA
e-mail: stuckerterika@hotmail.com

S.J. Stevens, M.D.
Department of Neurology, Hofstra North Shore—LIJ School of Medicine, Cushing Neuroscience Institute, 611 Northern Blvd, Suite 150, Great Neck, NY 11021, USA
e-mail: sstevens2@nshs.edu

Commentator: M. Sazgar, M.D. (✉)
University of California, Irvine Medical Center,
101 The City Drive South, Pavilion I, Bldg. 30, Suite 123,
Orange, CA 92868, USA
e-mail: msazgar@uci.edu

© Springer International Publishing Switzerland 2016
M. Sazgar, C.L. Harden (eds.), *Controversies in Caring for Women with Epilepsy*, DOI 10.1007/978-3-319-29170-3_3

I would start out by obtaining as much detail as possible regarding the patient's seizure semiology, including her subjective perception, possible aura prior to her focal seizure, followed by description and sequence of the events observed by witnesses.

To get a full picture, it is important to establish the types of her seizures and detailed semiology. If patient has a warning/aura prior to her event I would instruct her in safety measures, like alarming people surrounding her as well as educating her family members and friends in first aid. Furthermore, I would encourage her to start a seizure diary including monitoring her menstrual period pattern [1]. I would discuss with her the potential seizure triggers and epilepsy risk factors, including the significance of the female menstrual period and its hormonal fluctuations.

Given that her seizures are predictable and therefore likely to be captured, I would plan on obtaining a sleep-deprived EEG, may be a serial of sleep-deprived EEGs or have her admitted to EMU (Epilepsy Monitoring Unit). The long-term video-EEG recording will hopefully provide me with information regarding the seizure type, epileptogenic zone, and potential coexistent seizure types. If this patient meets criteria for possible pre-surgical evaluation, I would obtain an MRI of the brain with Epilepsy protocol. If MRI is negative, I would consider getting a PET scan or potentially a MEG scan if appropriate interictal discharges are present.

However while I am obtaining more information on her seizure type and potential surgical candidacy, I would discuss her medical treatment options. The optimal treatment option in this scenario is debatable and rather based on individual patient medical history and personal situation as well as personality type.

Hormone-associated seizures can often be predicted if patients keep a detailed log of their menstrual periods. Furthermore this opens up a potential of variable treatment options, including choosing low-dose-containing hormonal contraceptive versus progestin-only-containing contraceptive agent with the goal of regulating the seizures by regulating hormonal fluctuations. However side effects and tolerability need to be discussed.

In addition, the patient has an option of choosing medications on as-needed basis during her menstrual phase, like acetazolamide or clobazam [2].

Given the patient's age and that she is in a rather unpredictable period of life, like puberty, often characterized by frequent sleep deprivations, increased stress related to school, family, and friends, emotional instability, and hormonal fluctuations, one might decide to start an antiseizure medication, which will be continued through the years and be a good choice if the patient starts a family in the future. One of those medications is lamotrigine [3].

Despite the low frequency of her seizures, six times per year, I would be worried about the potential impact of the seizures on her memory and emotional state. I would explain the potential risks of frequent seizures causing sequelae to the brain as well as potential injuries due to dyscognitive features of her seizures.

Furthermore, I would discuss the requirements for driving restrictions after a seizure and go into more detailed discussion regarding seizure triggers like sleep deprivation, stress, noncompliance, infection, hormones, and interaction with other medications like antibiotics, antihistamines, and BCP.

Finally, depending on the findings on the video-EEG and Brain imaging, I would discuss with her the surgical options, which is the only cure in many cases.

AUTHOR #2'S RESPONSE

A 16-year-old woman with focal epilepsy having premenstrual focal seizures with dyscognitive features within 3 days of her menstrual period six times yearly should first be worked up similarly to other patients with epilepsy. If the patient was referred to an epilepsy center with such a history, her past medical records should first be obtained to prevent unnecessary repeat testing. The typical patient with this history who presents to an epilepsy center has likely already had MRI imaging and routine EEG testing performed by their general neurologist prior to the initial visit. With this in mind, ambulatory EEG or in-house video-EEG testing around the typical time of her seizures, at least 3 days prior to her menstrual period if she were to have a regular menstrual cycle, should be performed in order to assist in seizure characterization and localization.

In order to determine that the patient's seizures are consistently occurring within 3 days of her menstrual period, she should keep a seizure diary while undergoing treatment and evaluation. If it were found that her seizures clustered in alignment to her reproductive cycle, she would be labeled as having catamenial epilepsy [4]. This would be secondary to her natural cyclic variation in serum levels of estrogen and progesterone [4].

Two predominant patterns of catamenial seizures are seen during normal ovulatory cycles, perimenstrual (C1) and periovulatory (C2), with the perimenstrual pattern being more common. During the premenstrual period and during the days prior to ovulation there is a higher ratio of serum estradiol to progesterone, increasing the chance of seizure [4]. Furthermore, the rapid withdrawal of progesterone prior to menses may lead to an increase in seizure frequency at this time. A third pattern of catamenial seizures (C3) is seen in patients with inadequate luteal phase cycles and occurs less frequently than the other two patterns. Figure 3.1 illustrates these three patterns of catamenial epilepsy and how they are related to changes in estradiol and progesterone during the course of a typical reproductive cycle.

In a 16-year-old woman with perimenstrual catamenial epilepsy (C1 pattern), the first-line treatment should be anti-epileptic medications (AEDs). Since this is a 16-year-old female, valproate should be avoided because of the teratogenic risk and undesirable side-effect profile [5]. The potential side effects of increased appetite, weight gain, alopecia, polycystic ovary syndrome, and tremor would decrease acceptance in this population. Either lamotrigine or levetiracetam, newer medications possessing fewer undesirable side effects and a lower teratogenic risk, would be my first medication choices [5].

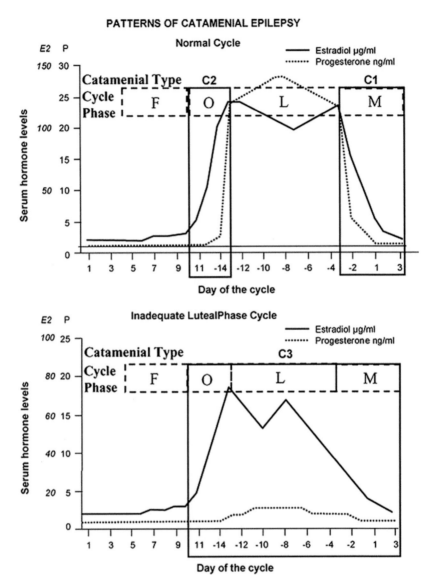

Fig. 3.1 Three patterns of catamenial epilepsy: perimenstrual (C1) and periovulatory (C2) exacerbations during normal ovulatory cycles and entire second half of the cycle (C3) exacerbation during inadequate luteal phase cycles. *F* follicular phase, *L* luteal phase, *M* menstruation, *O* ovulation (From Herzog AG. Catamenial epilepsy: definition, prevalence, pathophysiology, and treatment. Seizure. 2008;17:151–159 with permission)

Although AEDs are the first-line treatment for all patients with epilepsy, including those with catamenial epilepsy, adjunctive therapy with acetazolamide, benzodiazepines, and hormonal therapy may also be used. These treatments, which can be

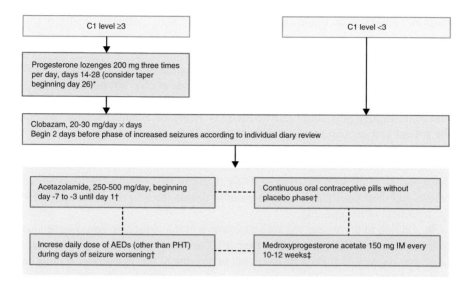

Fig. 3.2 Treatment algorithm for catamenial C1 (perimenstrual) pattern of seizures. Most treatments are for focal-onset seizures in women with regular menses. *C1 level 3* three times more seizures on days 25–3 compared with other days of the month, *AEDs* antiepileptic drugs, *PHT* phenytoin, *IM* intramuscularly. *If menses start before day 26, start dose tapering on that day according to the same pattern of decreases. †Widely undertaken but not supported by data from randomized, controlled trails. ‡Increased risk of osteoporosis and slow return to normal fertility (From Harden CL, Pennel PB. Neuroendocrine considerations in the treatment of men and women with epilepsy. Lancet Neurology 2013;12(1):72–83 with permission)

found in Fig. 3.2, are usually started during the second half of the menstrual cycle (days 14–26) for patients with catamenial C1 pattern of seizures.

A randomized double-blind, placebo-controlled multicenter clinical trial showed no benefit of natural progesterone as compared to placebo when grouping all patients with catamenial epilepsy together [6]. However, it was shown that progesterone was much more effective in patients with three or more seizures during the perimenstrual phase as compared to other days in the month [6]. If this patient were to have three or more seizures on days 25–3 of her menstrual cycle compared with the other days of the month, progesterone lozenges at 200 mg three times daily on days 14–28 could be used in addition to her AED therapy [6].

If the patient had less than three times the amount of seizures during the perimenstrual phase as compared to the rest of the month, or the patient had three or more seizures during this phase and failed AED plus progesterone combination therapy, clobazam adjunctive therapy could be used. Clobazam, at 20–30 mg/day for 10 days starting 2–4 days premenstrually, has been shown to reduce seizure frequency as compared to placebo [7].

If the patient failed the above treatment options, she could try intramuscular injections of medroxyprogesterone acetate, a synthetic progestin-only contraceptive agent, administered every 10–12 weeks, which been shown to decrease seizure frequency by 39 % at 1-year follow up in patients with catamenial epilepsy [8]. However, this agent has been shown to increase the risk of osteoporosis and brings about a slow return to normal fertility.

An increase in AEDs (other than phenytoin secondary to its nonlinear kinetics) during the days of worsening seizures, acetazolamide at 250–500 mg daily from 3 to 7 days prior to menses until day 1 of the menstrual cycle, or continuous use of oral contraceptive pills could also be tried [2]. However, it must be made clear to the patient and her parents that these three methods are commonly used in practice, but they are not supported by data from randomized, controlled trials. Additionally, prior to using any of the above options, the potential risks should be discussed in detail with the patient. Only then can the physician work with the patient and their family as a team in order to decide the best available option for the treatment of her epilepsy.

In addition to discussing the above treatment options, specific issues must also be brought up with this adolescent patient [9]. Pregnancy and contraception are two important issues which must be discussed in patients of this age group. It must be explained that many AEDs interact with oral contraceptive pills and that other forms of contraception may be needed. Additionally, since many teenage pregnancies are unplanned, teratogenic risks of prescribed AEDs and the need for folic acid supplementation should be discussed. Finally, state laws dealing with epilepsy and driving should be reviewed with this patient who is near or of driving age depending on the state in which she lives.

Reviewer's Comments

This is a case of a young lady with premenstrual catamenial epilepsy. Author #1 and Author #2 both suggest complete workup including consideration of admission to the video-EEG monitoring unit for seizure characterization and to determine therapeutic options such as surgical epilepsy candidacy. Both authors emphasize the importance of keeping a seizure diary in relation to menstrual cycle to establish the true catamenial epilepsy pattern. Author #1 prefers starting the patient on lamotrigine, and Author #2 suggests either lamotrigine or levetiracetam to begin with and trying to avoid valproate for its less favorable side-effect profile and teratogenicity.

Once the premenstrual catamenial nature of the patient's seizures is established (C1 pattern), both authors agree on trial of hormonal therapy. Author #2 points out the recent NIH-sponsored phase III clinical trial by Dr. Herzog et al. which found a subset of patients with premenstrual exacerbation of their seizures to respond to natural progesterone lozenges which certainly can be offered to this patient.

Both authors suggest other methods commonly used in practice but not supported by data from randomized controlled trials. These include temporary increase in AED dose, intramuscular injections of depot medroxyprogesterone acetate

(DMPA), oral contraceptives preferably progestin-only tablets or use of clobazam or acetazolamide premenstrually.

Finally the authors emphasize the importance of detailed counselling to the patient and family regarding lifestyle modifications, pregnancy, and implication of having uncontrolled epilepsy in driving privileges. In brief, there seems to be a general agreement of practitioners in the field of epilepsy of the steps they take in caring for young women with catamenial epilepsy.

Suggested Management

1. Establish true catamenial pattern of epilepsy by charting seizures and menstrual cycle
2. Consider progesterone lozenges/natural progesterone for C1 pattern
3. Consider synthetic progestin/or injections of DMPA
4. Consider acetazolamide 250 mg twice daily or 500 mg twice daily to be used around the 7–10 days of seizure exacerbation as determined by the seizure diary
5. Consider clobazam 20–30 mg divided twice a day or one dose at night for 10 days, starting 2 days prior and throughout the identified seizure exacerbation dates
6. Small increase in baseline AEDs about 2 days prior to the identified period of seizure exacerbation for up to 10 days. Be cautious about phenytoin, carbamazepine, or other medications with higher risk for toxicity
7. Counsel the patient regarding pregnancy, conception, driving, and seizure safety issues

References

1. Pennel PB. Pregnancy, epilepsy and women's issues. Continuum. 2013;19(3):697–714.
2. Harden CL, Pennel PB. Neuroendocrine considerations in the treatment of men and women with epilepsy. Lancet Neurol. 2013;12(1):72–83.
3. Tomson T, Battino D. Teratogenic effects of antiepileptic drugs. Lancet Neurol. 2012;11(9):803–13.
4. Herzog AG. Catamenial epilepsy: definition, prevalence, pathophysiology and treatment. Seizure. 2008;17:151–9.
5. Hernández-Díaz S, Smith CR, Shen A, et al. Comparative safety of antiepileptic drugs during pregnancy. Neurology. 2012;78(21):1692–9.
6. Herzog A, Fowler K, Smithson S, et al. Progesterone vs placebo therapy for women with epilepsy: a randomized clinical trial. Neurology. 2012;52:1959–66.
7. Feely M, Calvert R, Gibson J. Clobazam in catamenial epilepsy: a model for evaluating anticonvulsants. Lancet. 1982;2:71–3.
8. Mattson RH, Cramer JA, Caldwell BV, et al. Treatment of seizures with medroxyprogesterone acetate: preliminary report. Neurology. 1984;34:1255–8.
9. Appleton RE, Neville BG. Teenagers with epilepsy. Arch Dis Child. 1999;81:76–9.

Chapter 4
Contraception Choice in Adolescence

Barry E. Gidal, Mindl M. Messinger, and Katherine Noe

Case Scenario

An 18-year-old girl is a freshman in community college and has a history of focal epilepsy of left frontal origin due to cortical dysplasia. She is managed on oxcarbazepine and has remained seizure free in the past year. She informs you that she is sexually active and has been in stable relationship with her boyfriend in the past 6 months. She is asking you for advice on starting contraception. What form of contraception are you most likely to recommend to her? What will be your advice if she was on lamotrigine, topiramate, or levetiracetam?

B.E. Gidal, Pharm.D.
University of Wisconsin School of Pharmacy,
777 Highland Avenue, Madison, WI 53705, USA
e-mail: Barry.Gidal@wisc.edu

M.M. Messinger, Pharm.D.
Pharmacy Department, Texas Children's Hospital,
6621 Fannin St. Suite WB1120, Houston, TX 77030, USA
e-mail: mmmessin@texaschildrens.org

K. Noe, M.D., Ph.D.
Department of Neurology, Mayo Clinic Arizona,
5777 E. Mayo Blvd., Phoenix, AZ 85054, USA
e-mail: noe.katherine@mayo.edu

Commentator: C.L. Harden, M.D. (✉)
Mount Sinai Health System, Mount Sinai Beth Israel Phillips Ambulatory Care Center,
10 Union Square East, Suite 5D, New York, NY 10003, USA
e-mail: charden@chpnet.org

© Springer International Publishing Switzerland 2016
M. Sazgar, C.L. Harden (eds.), *Controversies in Caring for Women
with Epilepsy*, DOI 10.1007/978-3-319-29170-3_4

AUTHOR #1'S RESPONSE

Women of childbearing potential with epilepsy need accurate information about potential interactions between their anti-epileptic drug (AED) and hormonal contraceptives. Given the increased risk for fetal malformations and developmental disorders in children exposed to AEDs in the first trimester of pregnancy, is it particularly important that women with epilepsy have reliable contraception to minimize the risk of an unplanned pregnancy.

For all women, contraceptive choice should include consideration of effectiveness against unintended pregnancy and sexually transmitted disease, cost, safety, and what is acceptable to her and her partner. Choice may also be dictated by the timing of any planned future pregnancy. Amongst women aged 15–19 in the United States, condoms are the most popular form of contraceptive (96 % ever use), followed by oral contraceptive pills (OCPs) (56 %), depot medroxyprogesterone injections (20 %), contraceptive patch (10 %), and the vaginal ring (5 %) [1]. For women who do not desire pregnancy for several years, long-acting reversible contraceptives such as an intrauterine device (IUD) or implanted progesterone rods are also appropriate. Fewer than 5 % of young women in the United States use long-acting reversible contraception, but the rates are increasing [1]. For women with epilepsy, additional concerns include the potential for interactions between AED and hormonal contraceptives, as well as the potential for hormonal contraceptives to influence seizure control for better or worse. Coexisting medical conditions such as migraine headache may add further complexity to the choice of contraception.

For purposes of this discussion, I will assume our patient is able to be compliant with and has no contraindication (other than epilepsy) to any form of contraception felt appropriate, is not planning pregnancy in the near future, and is not intending to become abstinent. These are issues I clarify with patients in my practice as part of any dialogue about contraception.

Based on popularity and familiarity, many young women are interested in the oral pill for contraception. Oxcarbazepine, along with other hepatic cytochrome P450 inducing AEDs, can increase the metabolism of estrogens and progesterones in the liver (Table 4.1). This may result in loss of efficacy for OCPs (both combined estrogen/progesterone and progesterone-only pills), emergency contraception ("morning after pill"), the contraceptive patch, and the vaginal ring. The CDC guidelines on eligibility for contraceptive use recommend against these methods for women using enzyme-inducing AEDs [2]. There is similarly a potential interaction between these AEDs and the progesterone implant, although the level of risk is classified as lower [2]. Thus, for our case patient with epilepsy well controlled on oxcarbazepine, I would recommend an IUD as her most effective contraceptive choice. Past concerns that use of IUD in adolescents could lead to infertility or pelvic inflammatory disease have not proven true, and the device has been well tolerated in this age group [1]. Depot medroxyprogesterone injection (Depo-Provera) is another option, but is less favored due to the risk of weight gain and loss of bone mineral density.

Table 4.1 Antiepileptic
drugs that may reduce the
efficacy of hormonal
contraceptives

Carbamazepine
Eslicarbazepine
Felbamate
Oxcarbazepine
Perampanel[a]
Phenobarbital
Phenytoin
Primidone
Rufinamide
Topiramate[a]

[a]Effect seen at higher doses

There is also the option to consider changing her to a non-enzyme-inducing AED to facilitate a greater choice in hormonal contraceptive options. For example, if she was on Keppra she could effectively use the pill, the patch, the vaginal ring, or the implanted progesterone rod. Of these, as noted above, the combined OCP is the most frequently used prescription contraceptive in this age group in the United States, and is the most common contraceptive chosen by young women in my practice.

Topiramate at doses above 200 mg/day has similar interactions with hormonal contraceptive agents as oxcarbazepine. Therefore, if she was on higher dose topiramate therapy I would also recommend an IUD. Lower dose topiramate opens the door to use of the OCP, but I would counsel the patient to ensure she understands that this would no longer be effective if we had to increase the topiramate dose in the future.

If she was on lamotrigine, OCPs are an option, but there are specific challenges. Lamotrigine serum levels can be significantly reduced when used in conjunction with an OCP [3]. If unaddressed, this could result in breakthrough seizures. If this patient was stable on lamotrigine and wanted to start the oral birth control pill as her contraceptive of choice, I would recommend checking a serum lamotrigine level prior to initiation of the contraceptive, making an increase in her dose (30–50 % based on judgement) at the time the pill is started, then rechecking the serum level and fine tuning the lamotrigine dose as needed on week 2 or 3 of her active birth control pill. Theoretically women may experience an increased serum level of lamotrigine with associated signs and symptoms of toxicity during the week of placebo contraceptive pills when they experience withdrawal bleeding. In clinical practice, I have only very rarely encountered this issue; however, I do discuss the potential with my patients. If problematic, I would consider transitioning to an extended cycle OCP regimen where the placebo pills are not taken each month or transitioning to an alternative form of contraception. The patient should be reminded that if she discontinues the OCP, the dose of her lamotrigine should also be reduced to avoid elevated serum levels.

AUTHOR #2'S RESPONSE

In this case presented, our patient is asking for advice on contraception. Our objectives will be to discuss the most common options for contraception in this young woman, as well as to discuss special considerations based upon specific AED selection.

There are two general options of contraception, hormonal and non-hormonal. Hormonal contraceptives (HC) are available in oral formulations (combined OCP or progesterone-only), as well as non-oral formulations (patch, ring, implant, IUD containing progesterone, and progestogen injections). The non-hormonal contraceptives include copper IUDs or barrier methods, such as condoms and diaphragms. The efficacy of each agent, thus the failure rate (pregnancy per year per 100 women), is highly dependent on correct and consistent use [4]. While OCP failure rate is quite low in healthy women who are very adherent (~1 %), the failure rate in women with epilepsy is substantially higher (~3–6 %). Implants and IUDs are the most effective, followed by HC, while barrier methods are the least effective. See Table 4.2 for inclusive list. Women should discuss the risks and benefits of

Table 4.2 Pregnancy rate (percent) during first year of use of contraception (least effective to most effective)

Method	Typical use	Perfect use
No method	85	85
Spermicides	28	18
Fertility awareness-based methods	24	0.4–5
Withdrawal	22	4
Sponge		
Parous women	24	20
Nulliparous women	12	9
Condom		
Female	21	5
Male	18	2
Diaphragm	12	6
Combined pill and progestin-only pill	9	0.3
Evra patch	9	0.3
NuvaRing	9	0.3
Depo-Provera	6	0.2
IUDs		
Copper	0.8	0.6
Mirena (levonorgestrel intrauterine system)	0.2	0.2
Implant	0.05	0.05
Female sterilization	0.5	0.5
Male sterilization	0.15	0.1

Data refer to number of pregnancies per 100 women during first year of use
Adapted from Trussell J. Contraceptive failure in the United States. Contraception 2011; 83:397 with permission

each method with their gynecologist; reviewing such is beyond the scope of this section. Recall, only barrier methods protect against HIV or sexually transmitted infections [4].

HC contain estrogen and/or progestogen components, whose mechanism is inhibiting ovulation and fertilization. These products achieve contraception via the synergistic effects of progesterone and ethinyl estradiol (EE) on suppression of ovulation. While doses of EE needed to suppress ovulation would need to be in the range of 100 μg if given alone, substantially lower doses (20–30 μg) can be effective for cycle control when given in combination with a progestin. While most pharmacokinetic studies have focused on EE metabolism, it is important to recognize that it is the progestin component that is likely more important in preventing ovulation [5].

Unfortunately, both of these hormones (both EE and progestins) are extensively metabolized both in the gut and liver via cytochrome P450 (CYP450), particularly CYP3A4, thus are susceptible to drug interactions, particularly enzyme induction [4, 5]. In addition to increased first pass metabolism, enzyme induction can also result in increased production of sex hormone-binding globulin, which will ultimately reduce free or biologically active steroid concentrations. In this type of patient therefore, selection of an appropriate AED will include not only consideration of efficacy and adverse effects, but potential drug interactions as well.

Some of our commonly used AEDs, including both older traditional agents such as carbamazepine, phenytoin, and phenobarbital display the pharmacologic property of induction of both cytochrome P450 and UDP-glucuronyl transferase isozymes. This property of enzyme induction may also be seen (albeit to a lessor effect) for several of the newer generation agents including oxcarbazepine, eslicarbazepine, topiramate, felbamate, and possibly lamotrigine and perampanel. It is noteworthy that the induction of CYP3A4 for these newer agents appears to be dose-dependent. This would imply that at lower doses, one may not see a substantial kinetic effect, but that as AED dose is gradually titrated up over time, a new interaction could manifest.

For example, topiramate at doses greater than 200 mg/day may alter steroid concentrations, while doses below this might not. These enzyme-inducing AEDs (EIAEDs) have the potential to reduce the efficacy of HC by increasing steroid metabolism, and consequently reducing circulating hormone concentrations [5]. Should we elect to use topiramate in this patient, careful attention must be paid to final maintenance dose. It should also be recognized that these are average changes. It is possible that women receiving less than 200 mg/day might still display meaningful changes in plasma concentrations. This reduced efficacy is possible with most forms of HC [4, 6]. Therefore, patients treated with an EIAED and HC are at increased risk of contraceptive failure [6]. Limited data have shown a modest decrease in levonorgestrel with lamotrigine use, but without ovulation, therefore a very conservative approach would be to consider it an EIAED for contraceptive purposes [7].

In general OCP do not affect AED levels with the exception of lamotrigine [8]. The effect of OCP is to rapidly increase lamotrigine metabolism, resulting in potentially clinically meaningful declines (~50 %) in lamotrigine plasma concentrations. These effects can also dissipate quickly during the pill-free interval. Therefore, should we decide to use lamotrigine in this patient, plasma drug monitoring should be performed during days 7–21 of the cycle, as well as during the pill-free week [5].

There are two ways to tackle the contraceptive and EIAED interaction: (1) Use an AED that does not alter HC, or (2) use a contraception that does not undergo hepatic metabolism. This decision needs to be patient specific. Our case is of a patient who is seizure free on her current AED, thus switching AEDs may put her at risk of seizure recurrence. This is not optimal especially at her age, in college, and likely driving. On the other hand, had this been a patient with newly diagnosed epilepsy who was already on HC, starting an AED that would treat the seizure type without interacting with HC would be ideal. As for selection of non-inducing AED, drugs such as levetiracetam, lacosamide, or a gabapentinoid (e.g., gabapentin or pregabalin) would be reasonable considerations. Not only will these drugs not cause induction of the HC, the HC will likewise not interfere with any of these medications.

As part of our approach, we will also review the available contraceptive options for our patient and encourage her to discuss the risks and benefits of each with her gynecologist prior to making a decision. Oxcarbazepine is an EIAED, and can therefore reduce the efficacy of HC. Thinking not only in terms of drug interactions, but importantly individual contraceptive failure rates, the option with the lowest failure rate would be a copper IUD. Similarly, hormonal IUDs, such as Mirena®, act locally and therefore not considered affected by EIAEDs, but more data is needed.

Another potential approach would include Depo-Provera® (depot medroxyprogesterone acetate) an intramuscular injection administered every 12 weeks. Since EIAEDs can reduce the efficacy of progesterone, it is suggested to administer injections every 10 weeks [4], although this is controversial due to lack of studies. In addition, there is concern that this depot injection can result in reductions in bone mass, and a potential delay in return to fertility should she begin to consider starting a family.

The combined OCP is the most commonly used form of contraception, but efficacy has been shown to be reduced in women treated with AEDs [4, 5]. To overcome the reduced hormone levels, it is recommended by some to use a higher content of EE (50 µg as opposed to 20–30 µg). Women should monitor for breakthrough bleeding, and if occurs, a higher dose is recommended [4–6]. The limitation, however, is a lack of available products with this estrogen content. Again, it is important to remember that it is the progestin component that is likely most important for contraception. Another compensatory method is to omit the pill-free (or placebo) week and to continuously take the OCPs for 3–4 cycles, followed by a shorter, pill-free break of 4 days [7]. Both patients and clinicians may be concerned about adverse effects from increased exposure to hormones using these types of strategies. This is certainly a legitimate concern. It should also be recognized however that these potential problems are a result of increased plasma concentrations of the hormones, and that with the expected increased first pass metabolism from EIAEDs, these effects might be mitigated by reduced steroid bioavailability.

Despite these compensatory measures, HCs may still not provide full protection, thus a barrier method can be used in addition to help reduce the failure rate. The failure rate of EIAEDs with HC is still likely lower than if using barrier methods alone [5].

Unacceptable options include the progestogen-only products including pills [5] and the implant (Nexplanon®), which is contraindicated with EIAEDs due to high failure rates [4].

Women on AEDs must understand the potential for interactions between their AED and HC in order to ensure the best efficacy for both classes. Finally, regardless of ultimate AED choice, adherence to contraception must be emphasized. This is even more important should even a modest EIAED be employed.

Reviewer's Comments

Contraception in women with epilepsy taking AEDs is challenging since basically the patient wants to know "which form of contraception is best for me?" This is certainly not a one-size-fits-all answer, but authors both do an excellent job of outlining the issues of AED and hormonal contraception interactions with the medication our example patient is taking, oxcarbazepine, and discuss the options in the setting of taking other AEDs as well. Within these two documents, a good background of the landscape of contraception use in the United States is presented along with their usual failure rates (see Table 4.2). Further, a background on the mechanism of OCPs is provided by Author #2's contribution, which is always helpful to review and provides greater understanding of the appropriate contraceptive choice. Notably, the use of the progesterone-only pill as a contraception option for women taking lamotrigine is not endorsed in either review, due to the small but possibly clinically important effect of lamotrigine on increasing progesterone clearance and therefore permitting pregnancy.

Author #1 puts forth the opinion that the IUD should be offered to our example patient, a choice that many of us would endorse. Author #1 also points out that the current generation of IUDs does not carry the risks of the earlier versions and are highly effective. Both authors discuss the dose-related interactions with topiramate use, with Author #2 elegantly pointing out that "Should we elect to use topiramate in this patient, careful attention must be paid to final maintenance dose. It should also be recognized that these are average changes. It is possible that women receiving less than 200 mg/day might still display meaningful changes in plasma concentrations." Therefore, it is the unknown interindividual variability in drug interactions that leads us toward a more black-and-white approach. The overall message here is to avoid hormonal contraception in women taking AEDs with any risk of interaction with exogenous hormones and consider the IUD. Hormonal contraception is considered only for those women taking AEDs with no potential for interaction.

Suggested Management

1. Current thinking regarding contraception use in women with epilepsy taking AEDs is to avoid hormonal contraception in women taking AEDs that have any interaction effect on reproductive hormone metabolism, since the individual variability of the effect is broad and unpredictable.
2. The IUD remains an important mainstay of contraceptive options in the epilepsy population.

References

1. Ott MA, Sucato GS, Committee on Adolescence. Technical report: contraception for adolescents. Pediatrics. 2014;134:e1257–81.
2. Centers for Disease Control and Prevention. U.S. medical eligibility criteria for contraceptive use, 2010. MMWR Recomm Rep. 2010;59(RR04):1–86.
3. Sabers A, Ohman I, Christensens J, Tomson T. Oral contraceptives reduce lamotrigine plasma levels. Neurology. 2003;61(4):570–1.
4. Reddy DS. Clinical pharmacokinetic interactions between antiepileptic drugs and hormonal contraceptives. Exp Rev Clin Pharmacol. 2010;3(2):183–92.
5. Reimers A, Brodtkorb E, Sabers A. Interactions between hormonal contraception and antiepileptic drugs: clinical and mechanistic considerations. Seizure. 2015;28:66–70.
6. O'Brien MD, Guillebaud J. Contraception for women taking antiepileptic drugs. J Fam Plann Reprod Health Care. 2010;36(4):239–42.
7. Johnston CA, Crawford PM. Anti-epileptic drugs and hormonal treatments. Curr Treat Options Neurol. 2014;16(5):288.
8. Crawford P. Best practice guidelines for the management of women with epilepsy. Epilepsia. 2005;46 Suppl 9:117–24.

Part II
Pre-Conception Counseling

Chapter 5
Folic Acid Supplementation

Kaarkuzhali Babu Krishnamurthy and George Lee Morris III

Case Scenario

A 26-year-old woman is taking valproic acid for her stable Juvenile Myoclonic Epilepsy. There has been no other seizure medication which controlled her convulsive seizures except for valproic acid. She is taking prenatal vitamins since she is sexually active. Would you recommend higher dose of folic acid to her? How would you counsel her regarding the evidence for the dose you are recommending? Would it change your management if she was taking lamotrigine, topiramate, or levetiracetam?

K.B. Krishnamurthy, B.S.E.E., M.D.
Director, Women's Health in Epilepsy, Co-chair, Ethics Advisory Committee,
Department of Neurology, Beth Israel Deaconess Medical Center,
330 Brookline Avenue, East/Kirstein 457, Boston, MA 02215, USA
e-mail: bkrishna@bidmc.harvard.edu

G.L. Morris III, M.D.
Aurora Health Care, St. Luke's Medical Center, Milwaukee, WI, USA

Center for Urban Population Health, Milwaukee, WI, USA

Zilber School of Public Health, Milwaukee, WI, USA

UW School of Public Health and Medicine, UW-Madison, Madison, WI, USA

Marquette University, Milwaukee, WI, USA

Epilepsy Center, St. Luke's Medical Center,
Suite 570, 2801 KK River Parkway, Milwaukee, WI 53211, USA
e-mail: George.Morris@aurora.org

Commentator: M. Sazgar, M.D. (✉)
University of California, Irvine Medical Center,
101 The City Drive South, Pavilion I, Bldg. 30, Suite 123, Orange, CA 92868, USA
e-mail: msazgar@uci.edu

© Springer International Publishing Switzerland 2016
M. Sazgar, C.L. Harden (eds.), *Controversies in Caring for Women
with Epilepsy*, DOI 10.1007/978-3-319-29170-3_5

AUTHOR #1'S RESPONSE

In caring for a woman of childbearing potential with juvenile myoclonic epilepsy, for whom only valproic acid (VPA) has provided complete seizure control, due care and consideration must be given to preconception counseling, particularly with respect to modifiable risk factors. Presuming that the lowest dose of VPA) necessary to provide seizure control is in use, and the patient understands the risks of major congenital malformations related to VPA, a recommendation for the use of folic acid may provide added risk reduction during pregnancy. However, there is no consensus opinion as to the optimal dosing of folic acid in women with epilepsy (WWE) [1].

The Centers for Disease Control (CDC) and US Public Health Service (USPHS) recommend that women of childbearing potential use 0.4 mg of oral folic acid daily to prevent neural tube defects [2]. While this recommendation is independent of the presence of other health considerations, it provides a lower limit for the recommended daily dosing of folate for patients with epilepsy. Likewise, for women who have already had one pregnancy involving a neural tube deficiency, the USPHS recommendation is for use of 4 mg of folic acid per day in order to reduce the recurrence risk during subsequent pregnancies [3]. This may then provide the upper limit of our recommendation for WWE.

There is no significant evidence that folate exposure causes problems for people with epilepsy. While folate supplementation may lower plasma phenytoin levels, this known interaction can be monitored for with dosing of phenytoin correspondingly adjusted. Thus, the risk associated with folate supplementation for WWE seems low in comparison to the potential benefit, so recommending daily dosing of folic acid while in the childbearing years would be warranted. The optimal dose, however, remains in question, even after an extensive analysis of the available literature provided by the major professional organization for epileptologists [1].

Many studies have confirmed that VPA use in pregnancy is associated with a higher risk of major congenital malformations, including neural tube defects. The mechanism of this process is incompletely understood, although there is evidence that both plasma and red cell folate levels are decreased in the presence of intercurrent VPA use [4]. In chick eggs, the teratogenic effects of VPA administration can be lessened by the co-administration of folic acid [5]. Whereas a double-blind, randomized-controlled trial comparing the rates of neural tube pregnancies in women taking VPA with or without use of folic acid would be unethical, observational studies have shown mild evidence of a protective effect of folic acid [Jentink] in WWE taking VPA. Thus, particularly in WWE taking VPA, the evidence seems clearly to weigh in favor of folic acid supplementation.

Given that one specific result of VPA exposure is a higher risk of neural tube defects in utero, and there is evidence to support a reduced risk of neural tube defects after higher dose folate supplementation in women who have already had one neural tube pregnancy, I typically recommend use of 4 mg of folic acid per day in WWE taking valproic acid.

For patients on lamotrigine, topiramate, or levetiracetam, there does not seem to be an increased risk specifically for neural tube defects, nor is there significant evidence to support lowered serum or red cell folate levels in women taking these medications. With use of these medications, therefore, I would recommend only the standard 1 mg of oral folic acid per day.

As an added consideration, I maintain patients on the "pregnancy" doses of folic acid throughout their childbearing years. While some practitioners may adhere more rigorously to the CDC and USPHS guidelines, only increasing the folic acid dose in anticipation of pregnancy, the relatively high likelihood of unplanned pregnancies (estimated to be 50 % in some studies), may result in women may be unaware of a pregnancy until past the point of neural tube closure (approximately 6 weeks gestational age). This is particularly true in WWE who may have coincident reproductive endocrine dysfunction, resulting in unpredictable or irregular cycles. The beneficial effect of folic acid administration occurs prior to and during the period of neurulation, so it would be easy to miss the opportunity to have women take the vitamin early in pregnancy if not given on a regular basis, whether or not pregnancy is contemplated.

In summary, for our patient taking VPA regularly, with effective seizure control, I would recommend that she take 4 mg of folic acid daily throughout her childbearing years. For patients taking lamotrigine, topiramate, or levetiracetam, I would recommend 1 mg of folate per day. I would take the added precaution of providing the patient with a prescription for the appropriate dose of folic acid along with prescriptions for the anticonvulsant medication, to emphasize the importance of adherence to the vitamin supplement.

AUTHOR #2'S RESPONSE

The use of folic acid during pregnancy for the reduction of neural tube defects was established and recommendations for a dose of 0.4 mg of folate in otherwise healthy women was made by the Medical Research Council (MRC) based on a review of the literature showing double-blinded evidence of a reduction [6]. This MRC guideline recommended higher doses of 4 mg for at-risk groups including those on antiepileptic drugs. The evidence suggesting value to higher doses came from the work of Wald in 2001 showing a relationship between dose and the incidence of neural tube defects was sustained to a plasma concentration of 9 ng/mL and had recommended 5 mg doses based on this observation [7].

A 2003 Practice Bulletin from the American College of Obstetrics and Gynecology recommended the 4 mg daily folate dose noting that it reduced neural tube defects 82 % but conceding that the mechanism by which antiepileptic drugs produce neural tube defects may be different specifically referencing valproic acid in this advisory [8]. The report referred to the 1991 recommendation of the Center for Disease Control recommendation of a daily 4 mg ingestion of folate and that the

US Public Health Service had recommended a 0.4 mg daily folate dose which the American College of Obstetrics and Gynecology had endorsed the following year. The report emphasized the preconception use of 0.4 mg of folate which could be found in over-the-counter multivitamins.

A Practice Parameter update from the American Academy of Neurology and American Epilepsy Society concluded that evidence for supplementation of 0.4 mg of daily folate was supported by Class C evidence [9]. There were some Class III studies supporting a reduction in major congenital malformations but some that showed no effect. Preconception use of folate was recommended by this report. This report found insufficient evidence to recommend higher doses of 4 or 5 mg of folate daily. This report suggests there is no currently known evidence of harm with folate supplementation in these higher doses.

Our 26-year-old woman is being treated with valproic acid for stable Juvenile Myoclonic Epilepsy. The case further states that no other seizure medications have controlled her tonic-clonic events. One option presented is the possible conversion to other antiepileptic medications, lamotrigine, topiramate, or levetiracetam which have all had reported success in treating myoclonus and tonic-clonic seizures. The sentence suggests that no other drug has successfully treated her convulsions and anecdotal reports of the risk of convulsions during conception and the risk to mother would appear to support no conversion if all three of these agents were unsuccessful.

First, a strong recommendation of effective birth control should be a mandate. Appropriate timing for her conception and possible adjustment of the valproic acid dose to the lowest effective level would be advisable. A recent publication by Baker et al. has suggested that cognitive development in children exposed to valproate in utero is slowed when compared to children exposed to other antiepileptic drugs but less so when the dose was less than 800 mg. This report references another study showing a dose-dependent effect on major congenital malformations with increasing doses of valproic acid. This dose-dependency is seen in other antiepileptic medications so finding the lowest optimal dose of any antiepileptic medication would be important [10].

The evidence supports having this woman continue taking her perinatal vitamins with the 0.4 mg of folate. The evidence does not argue against the higher doses of 4 or 5 mg of folate daily with theoretical but no proven benefit and with no clear adverse effect from the higher doses of folate.

Reviewer's Comments

As pointed out by both Author #1 and Author #2, folic acid deficiency can increase the risk of neural tube defects. Folic acid supplementation is recommended for WWE who are planning pregnancy as it is for all women of childbearing age when not using contraception. Some AEDs such as valproic acid, carbamazepine, phenobarbital, phenytoin, and primidone alter folic acid metabolism and may decrease its levels in the blood. The effective dose of folic acid is a matter of debate and there is insufficient data for clear advice regarding the dose.

Author #2 refers to a systematic review by Wald et al. which concluded 5 mg per day of folic acid in women without epilepsy renders 85 % protection against neural tube defects [7, 11]. He also points out the MRC guideline recommending higher doses of 4 mg folic acid supplementation for at-risk groups including those on anti-epileptic drugs. He concludes his discussion stating that "evidence does not argue against the higher doses of 4 or 5 mg of folate daily with theoretical but no proven benefit and with no clear adverse effect from the higher doses of folate."

Author #2 also advocates for higher 4 mg dose of folic acid supplementation in WWE who take valproic acid based on the fact that VPA results in higher risk for major congenital malformation and neural tube defects.

Suggested Management

1. The recommended dose of folic acid by American Academy of Neurology is a minimum of 0.4 mg folic acid supplementation daily prior to conception and throughout the pregnancy in WWE [10].
2. A dose of 4–5 mg daily folic acid in women taking carbamazepine, phenobarbital, phenytoin, primidone, and valproic acid is common practice due to higher risk for folate deficiency and neural tube defects.

References

1. Harden CL, et al. Management issues for women with epilepsy—focus on pregnancy (an evidence-based review): III. Vitamin K, folic acid, blood levels, and breast feeding. Report of the Quality Standards Subcommittee and Therapeutics and Technology Assessment Subcommittee of the American Academy of Neurology and the American Epilepsy Society. Epilepsia. 2009;50(5):1247–55.
2. Centers for Disease Control. Effectiveness in disease and injury prevention use of folic acid for prevention of spina bifida and other neural tube defects—1983-1991. MMWR Morb Mortal Wkly Rep. 1991;40(30):513–6.
3. Centers for Disease Control. Recommendations for the use of folic acid to reduce the number of cases of spina bifida and other neural tube defects. MMWR Recomm Rep. 1992;41(RR-14):1–7.
4. Gidal BE, et al. Blood homocysteine, folate and vitamin B12 concentrations in patients with epilepsy receiving lamotrigine or sodium valproate for initial monotherapy. Epilepsy Res. 2005;64:161–6.
5. Umur AS, et al. Simultaneous folate intake may prevent adverse effect of valproic acid on neurulating nervous system. Childs Nerv Syst. 2012;28:729–37.
6. MRC Vitamin Study Research Group. Prevention of neural tube defects: results of the Medical Research Council Vitamin Study. Lancet. 1991;338:131.
7. Wald NJ, et al. Quantifying the effect of folic acid. Lancet. 2001;358:2069–73.

8. ACOG Committee on Bulletin. ACOG practice bulletin. Clinical management guidelines for obstetricians and gynecologists. Obstet Gynecol. 2003;102:203–13.
9. Harden CL, et al. Practice parameter update: management issues for women with epilepsy—focus on pregnancy (an evidence-based review): vitamin K blood levels, and breastfeeding. Neurology. 2009;73:142–9.
10. Baker GA, et al. IQ at 6 years after in utero exposure to antiepileptic drugs. Neurology. 2014;84:382–90.
11. Wald NJ, Hackshaw AD, Stone R, Sourial NA. Blood folic acid and vitamin B12 in relation to neural tube defects. Br J Obstet Gynaecol. 1996;103:319–24.

Chapter 6
Risk of Seizure During Pregnancy

Ajith Cherian, John C. DeToledo, Sahawat Tantikittichaikul,
and Sanjeev V. Thomas

Case Scenario

A 28-year-old woman presents to your office for consultation. She has been married
for 2 years and is planning to start a family and become pregnant. She is diagnosed
with partial epilepsy of temporal lobe origin 5 years ago and her seizures are controlled on lamotrigine 100 mg twice daily with no recurrence in the last year. She is
worried about the risk of seizure medications to her baby should she become pregnant. She wants to stop taking lamotrigine during her pregnancy. How do you counsel her regarding the risk of seizure recurrence during pregnancy and potential
seizure-related complications for her future pregnancy?

A. Cherian, M.D., D.M. post doctoral fellow (Epilepsy) • S.V. Thomas, M.D., D.M.
Department of Neurology, Sree Chitra Institute of Medical Sciences and Technology, Medical
College P.O., Trivandrum 695001, Kerala, India
e-mail: drajithcherian@yahoo.com; sanjeev.v.thomas@gmail.com

J.C. DeToledo, M.D. • S. Tantikittichaikul, M.D.
Department of Neurology, Texas Tech University Health Sciences Center School of Medicine,
3601 4th Street, STOP 8321, Lubbock, TX 79430, USA
e-mail: john.detoledo@ttuhsc.edu; s.tantikittichaikul@ttuhsc.edu

Commentator: C.L. Harden, M.D. (✉)
Mount Sinai Health System, Mount Sinai Beth Israel Phillips Ambulatory Care Center,
10 Union Square East, Suite 5D, New York, NY 10003, USA
e-mail:charden@chpnet.org

© Springer International Publishing Switzerland 2016   45
M. Sazgar, C.L. Harden (eds.), *Controversies in Caring for Women
with Epilepsy*, DOI 10.1007/978-3-319-29170-3_6

AUTHOR #1'S RESPONSE

Introduction and Conception Plan

This patient may be reassured by the fact that seizures and epilepsy affect 1/200 women of childbearing age and 0.5 % of all pregnancies occur in women with epilepsy. By no means is our patient alone and each year more than 20,000 children are born to women with epilepsy. Because this is common, a conception plan should be part of the management of all women with epilepsy who are of child-bearing age. Our patient is clearly apprehensive about possible undesirable outcomes that can be associated with epilepsy and the use of antiepileptic medications. If the type of epilepsy has a high recurrent rate without antiepileptic drug (AED), as in this case, continuation of AED should be encouraged for several reasons. As part of the visit, it often helps to remind patients and families that most women who have epilepsy deliver healthy babies. It can also be helpful to educate the patient of what she can do to help, specifically, adhering to folic acid supplementation and avoid having seizures. Smoking adds to the risk of premature contraction and preterm labor in WWE who take AED and if our patient is a smoker, she should be strongly encouraged to quit.

Epilepsy itself (even without treatment) can cause a slight increase in the risk of fetal malformation. Having uncontrolled seizures during the pregnancy also increases the risk for both mother and baby. By avoiding the more teratogenic drugs and giving adequate supplementation of folic acid and vitamin B12, the risk of major fetal malformations can be reduced to less than 5 % which is acceptable when we consider that uncontrolled seizures can increase the risk of small for gestational age, lower the verbal IQ of the offspring, increase risk of delivery complications and maternal death [1].

AED and Teratogenicity

AED have a class effect for increasing the risk of congenital anomalies (CA) such as neural tube defect, oral cleft, and cardiac anomalies. The risk is much higher with exposure in the first trimester, but some drugs, particularly valproic acid, can result in cognitive deficits even with exposure as late as the third trimester of pregnancy. Choice of AED and dosage are the very important in management of individual risks from epilepsy. Valproate has the highest risk of CA among the other AEDs [2]. Lamotrigine, oxcarbazepine, and levetiracetam seem to have the most favorable profiles. Nevertheless, they still increase the risk of oral cleft and neural tube defect respectively. The use of monotherapy and lower dose of AEDS are generally associated with lower risk of CA.

The relationship between dosage of AED and risk of CA raise some interesting questions (Fig. 6.1) [2]. This data suggests that low doses of less safe AEDs may carry a lower risk of CA than high doses of safer drugs. In Fig. 6.1, there is a suggestion that doses of valproic acid lower than 600 mg daily might be no worse

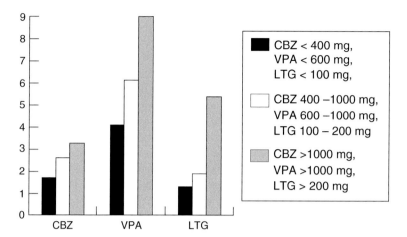

Fig. 6.1 Major congenital malformation rate (%) by drug dose. *CBZ* carbamazepine, *LTG* lamotrigine, *VPA* valproate (From J Morrow, A Russell, E Guthrie, L Parsons, I Robertson, R Waddell, B Irwin, R C McGivern, P J Morrison, and J Craig. Malformation risks of antiepileptic drugs in pregnancy: a prospective study from the UK Epilepsy and Pregnancy Register. J Neurol Neurosurg Psychiatry. 2006; 77(2): 193–198 with permission)

than higher doses of lamotrigine. This observation highlights an important aspect in the management of pregnant WWE—sometimes the treating physician has to use the AED that works best for a given patient. Having to use very high doses of a "safer" AED to control seizures that were controlled on much lower doses of a "less safe" AED is not necessarily safer for the fetus.

Predicting Risk of Recurrent Seizure During Pregnancy

Whereas pregnancy by itself does not seem to affect seizure frequency, there are a number of factors that coexist with the pregnancy that can increase the risk for seizures in WWE. Fear of medication side effects may decrease treatment compliance and is preventable by education and reassuring. Degree of seizure control prior to pregnancy is a reasonable predictor of risk of seizure recurrence during pregnancy where 80–90 % of WWE who were seizure free for 1 year prior to pregnancy will remain seizure free throughout the pregnancy [3]. Not all drugs are affected equally by pregnancy and understanding these changes in the metabolism and making the necessary adjustments is an important part of the seizure management in these cases.

Supplement for Pregnancy

Folic acid supplement with at least 0.4 mg but up to 4 mg/day in higher situations of higher risk is recommended before starting pregnancy. Adding vitamin B12 to the folic acid may confer some additional protection against spina bifida.

During Pregnancy

Lamotrigine is metabolized primarily via glucuronidation. Glucuronidation is a ubiquitous process found in all major body organs. The mature placenta has increased glucuronide conjugation that incrementally increases the elimination of lamotrigine after the second trimester of pregnancy. The American Academy of Neurology (AAN) recommends monitoring of lamotrigine level during pregnancy [4]. Levels of lamotrigine should be checked every trimester and whenever possible, levels should be maintained at the same range as before pregnancy. WWE taking AED during pregnancy have increased risk of obstetric complications but these risks are relatively small. These risks include pre-eclampsia and eclampsia, gestational hypertension, vaginal bleeding in late pregnancy, and preterm labor [5].

Postpartum Period

From mid-gestation onward, the placenta plays an important role in the metabolism and disposition of drugs both through oxidation and glucuronidation. Whereas not all P450 isoforms and glucuronidation pathways are equally affected, the activity of some enzymatic subsets can be induced by as much as 150 fold. Lamotrigine is metabolized by uridine glucuronosyl transferase (UGT) 1A3 and UGT1A4 and the activities of both are significantly increased in the mature placenta. With the abrupt elimination of this metabolic path for the lamotrigine by the removal of the placenta, the level of lamotrigine will show an abrupt increase that can be detected within hours to days after delivery. Reduction of the lamotrigine dose is generally recommended over a period of 2 weeks after delivery. Given the fact that 100 mg twice daily gave this patient complete control of her seizures, increasing her daily dose slightly by approximately 20–250 mg daily is suggested in order to compensate for inevitable triggers such as postpartum fatigue and sleep deprivation.

Conclusion

Our patient is not alone. She faces a decision faced by thousands of other WWE each year and with proper management, most will deliver healthy babies. She is already taking lamotrigine, an AED with extensive track record of better safety in pregnancy. Her seizures have been controlled with relatively low dose monotherapy for 1 year and she is tolerating this dose without side effects. With reassurance and folic acid supplementation, she will be in the lowest risk of CA group we have. Because her seizure type has a high risk for reoccurrence when AEDs are discontinued, she should be encouraged to continue her AED regime as the risk of complications from having seizures during her pregnancy may outweigh any benefits she might have by trying to go through pregnancy without proper treatment for her seizures.

AUTHOR #2'S RESPONSE

Introduction

The effect of pregnancy on seizure frequency is variable. Women with epilepsy are concerned whether seizures might worsen during pregnancy. Although it might seem ideal to withdraw AEDs during pregnancy, for most women this is not a realistic option.

Evidence Base

Will Seizures Cause Harm to Pregnancy?

A population-based retrospective study with secondary data from Taiwan had shown that women who had seizures during pregnancy had higher risk of babies with low birth weight, preterm or small for gestational age [6]. However a population-based study from Norway did not demonstrate such a difference [7]. A single brief tonic-clonic seizure has been shown to cause depression of the fetal heart rate for more than 20 min, and longer or repetitive tonic-clonic seizures are incrementally more hazardous to the fetus as well as the mother [8]. Major seizures can cause trauma that can result in rupture of fetal membranes leading to increased risk of infection, premature labor, and even fetal death.

What Is the Seizure Risk During Pregnancy?

The International multicenter EURAP registry had shown that women had remained seizure free in 58.3 % of the 1956 pregnancies that were followed up prospectively. Compared to first trimester of pregnancy, seizures remained unchanged for 63.6 %, worsened for 17.3 % and improved for 15.9 % during the second and third trimester. Status epilepticus though rare occurred in 1.8 % cases [9]. Modifiable factors like sleep deprivation, drug noncompliance, or substantial drop in blood levels of AEDs accounted for the increase in seizures in about 70 % women. The risk of seizure recurrence in pregnancy is higher in the second and third trimester of pregnancy and highest in the peripartum period. The data from Kerala Registry indicated that those who had seizures either due to localization-related epilepsy or in the pre-pregnancy month had significantly higher risk of recurrence of seizures during pregnancy [10]. With regard to risk of seizure recurrence during pregnancy and AED therapy, the EURAP data indicated that those who were on polytherapy or treatment with oxcarbazepine (OXC) were at higher risk of recurrence of seizures. The data on 1111 pregnancies on monotherapy from the Australian pregnancy registry showed that women who were on levetiracetam (LVT) had control of seizures comparable to those on carbamazepine or valproate which was better than those on lamotrigine (LTG) or topiramate [11]. A larger series from EURAP has confirmed that compared to other monotherapies, women on LTG are less likely to remain seizure free (58 %, $p=0.0001$) had more GTCS (21 %, $p<0.0001$) and higher risk of seizure worsening (20 % $p<0.01$) in spite of some degree of dose escalation or addition of second drug [12].

What Is the Specific Risk of Seizure Recurrence During Pregnancy for LTG?

Pharmacokinetics of AEDs demonstrates considerable variation between women and in between pregnancies in the same woman. There was a remarkable increase in the clearance of LTG and LVT (191 % and 207 %, respectively) during pregnancy and the blood levels may drop to less than 35 % from preconception baseline, which was associated with increased seizure risk [13]. The serum LTG concentration will begin to decrease within the first trimester and will reach its lowest concentration by mid-third trimester. The blood levels of LTG often rise after delivery, leading to symptoms of toxicity. LTG is metabolized primarily through the liver by glucuronidation. The genetic polymorphism of Uridine diphosphate (UDP) glucuronosyltransferase 1A4 (UGTIA4) is considered to be one of the main reasons for individual diversity of LTG kinetics during pregnancy.

Will Monitoring the Blood Level of AEDs Improve the Seizure Control During Pregnancy?

There is no uniformity in the recommendations between different guidelines with regard to monitoring of blood levels of AEDs during pregnancy. Seizure frequency during pregnancy increased when the LTG level decreased to 65 % of the preconception-individualized target LTG concentration. Serum monitoring of LTG, OXC, carbamazepine, phenytoin, and LEV have been advocated [4].

What Is the Risk of Fetal Malformations with LTG Exposure?

The North American AED Pregnancy Registry had reported birth defects in 15 new borns (five with cleft palate) out of 564 pregnancies on LTG monotherapy. Data from this registry later on pointed to higher risk of facial cleft (2.5 per thousand) when compared to population risk (0.37/1000) [14]. The UK Epilepsy and Pregnancy

Registry found 3.2 % of major malformations from pregnancies on LTG; however there was no excess risk of facial clefts [2]. The association between LTG exposure and fetal malformation appears to be dose dependent. Pregnancies exposed to LTG doses above 200 mg resulted in major congenital malformations in 5.4 % pregnancies [2]. The malformations frequently reported with LTG monotherapy are esophageal malformation, cleft palate, and club foot [15].

Counselling Points

- Seizures can aggravate in about 20 % of women with epilepsy during pregnancy
- Risk of seizure recurrence is more with LTG compared to certain other AEDs
- Seizures during pregnancy can adversely affect pregnancy and infant
- One should aim for optimal control of seizures at least effective dosage

Recommendations

1. It is important to reassure that most women with epilepsy would have safe pregnancy and healthy children.
2. The AAN guidelines state that there is good evidence in favor of monitoring blood levels of LTG, CBZ, and PHT during pregnancy while the evidence is only weak with regard to LEV and OXC.
3. Establish pre-pregnancy blood level for LTG.
4. Be prepared to escalate the AED dosage to match the pre-pregnancy levels in the second or third trimester and reduce the dosage in the postpartum if the dosage was increased during pregnancy.
5. One should start with folate supplementation in pre-pregnancy stage and continue through pregnancy and call for anomaly scans and other screening for malformations towards the end of first trimester.

The current literature indicates that this 28-year-old lady with temporal lobe epilepsy has a low risk of recurrence of seizures during pregnancy as she is on monotherapy and did not have any seizures in the past 1 year. Withdrawing the AEDs at this stage carries a significant risk of seizure relapse during pregnancy with all its accompanying hazards. It would be helpful to establish her pre-pregnancy blood level of lamotrigine which could serve as a baseline target level to be maintained during her pregnancy. The dosage of lamotrigine may have to be escalated in the second and third trimesters of pregnancy if the levels drop significantly. Any dose escalation in the last trimester may have to be reversed soon after delivery. I would also recommend that she maintain regular follow-up with her gynecologist and arrange to get detailed anomaly scan at 16 weeks of pregnancy.

Reviewer's Comments

These two authors have covered the entire scope of lamotrigine use during pregnancy, including the risks of its use during pregnancy, metabolism in detail, the use of blood levels, and the risks of seizures during pregnancy. Author #1 emphasized the importance of maintaining the lowest possible AED dose, yet following and maintaining the lamotrigine level through dose adjustment during pregnancy, since the decrease in levels does permit seizures. The explanation of the placental metabolism of lamotrigine is important as it reminds us that the lamotrigine levels will abruptly rise after birth with the delivery of this metabolic organ, and patients may quickly become lamotrigine toxic. Author #2 emphasized the risk of seizures themselves to the pregnancy, and raised another critical management point which is good sleep hygiene for this at-risk population. Author #2 also provided a wonderful overview of the expectations of the course of seizure occurrence across pregnancy based on current, high-quality literature. Both have arrived at the same conclusion after providing us with very different approaches to doing so, which is that this woman should continue taking her lamotrigine. Both authors stated that lamotrigine levels are integral for the management of this patient before, during, and after pregnancy. So a question can be raised from this—should lamotrigine be used during pregnancy if levels are not readily available? The increased risk of seizures with lamotrigine use during pregnancy, which presumably associates with not staying ahead of declining levels in many cases, alters the risk to benefit ratio of lamotrigine during pregnancy. While I agree with the management bullets put forth by Author #2 and really have nothing to add, we should ask ourselves as a community if we are not doing a disservice to stand behind lamotrigine use for its low teratogenicity but not also insist on the availability of levels when used during pregnancy so that the risk of seizures is also properly managed.

Suggested Management

1. When counselling the patient with epilepsy who wants to become pregnant, explain the potential risks of seizures to her and her fetus and how the benefits of seizure control by certain medications may outweigh the potentially teratogenic side effects.
2. Obtain baseline lamotrigine levels in all women of childbearing age with epilepsy taking this medication; use this as the therapeutic baseline level. Instruct them to call you as soon as they find out about pregnancy.
3. Consider obtaining monthly lamotrigine trough levels throughout pregnancy and more frequently if the levels are decreasing in order to maintain the therapeutic baseline level.
4. Adjust the dose of lamotrigine if the patient has seizure recurrence or preventatively if there has been a 25 % decrease in levels compared to her baseline.
5. Consider reducing the dose of lamotrigine back to pre-partum dose within 3 weeks of delivery. This dose reduction may need to begin within days of delivery if symptoms of lamotrigine toxicity occur.
6. Use daily folic acid supplementation in all women of childbearing age.

References

1. Harden CL, Meador KJ, Pennell PB, Hauser WA, Gronseth GS, French JA, et al. Practice parameter update: management issues for women with epilepsy—focus on pregnancy (an evidence-based review): teratogenesis and perinatal outcomes: report of the Quality Standards Subcommittee and Therapeutics and Technology Assessment Subcommittee. Neurology. 2009;73(2):133–41.
2. Morrow J, Russell A, Guthrie E, Parsons L, Robertson I, Waddell R, Irwin B, McGivern RC, Morrison PJ, Craig J. Malformation risks of antiepileptic drugs in pregnancy: a prospective study from the UK Epilepsy and Pregnancy Register. J Neurol Neurosurg Psychiatry. 2006;77(2):193–8.
3. Harden CL, Hopp J, Ting TY, Pennell PB, French JA, Hauser WA, et al. Practice parameter update: management issues for women with epilepsy—focus on pregnancy (an evidence-based review): obstetrical complications and change in seizure frequency: report of the Quality Standards Subcommittee and Therapeutics and Technology Assessment Subcommittee. Neurology. 2009;73(2):126–32.
4. Harden CL, Pennell PB, Koppel BS, Hovinga CA, Gidal B, Meador KJ, et al. Practice parameter update: management issues for women with epilepsy—focus on pregnancy (an evidence-based review): vitamin K, folic acid, blood levels, and breastfeeding: report of the Quality Standards Subcommittee and Therapeutics and Technology Assessment Subcommittee. Neurology. 2009;73(2):142–9.
5. Borthen I, Eide MG, Veiby G, Daltveit AK, Gilhus NE. Complications during pregnancy in women with epilepsy: population-based cohort study. BJOG. 2009;116(13):1736–42.
6. Chen YH, Chiou HY, Lin HC, Lin HL. Affect of seizures during gestation on pregnancy outcomes in women with epilepsy. Arch Neurol. 2009;66(8):979–84.
7. Borthen I, Eide MG, Daltveit AK, Gilhus NE. Obstetric outcome in women with epilepsy: a hospital-based, retrospective study. BJOG. 2011;118(8):956–65.
8. Teramo K, Hiilesmaa V, Bardy A, et al. Fetal heart rate during a maternal grand mal epileptic seizure. J Perinat Med. 1979;7:3–5.
9. EURAP Study Group. Seizure control and treatment in pregnancy: observations from the EURAP epilepsy pregnancy registry. Neurology. 2006;66(3):354–60.
10. Thomas SV, Syam U, Devi JS. Predictors of seizures during pregnancy in women with epilepsy. Epilepsia. 2012;53:e85–8.
11. Vajda FJ, O'Brien T, Lander C, Graham J, Eadie M. The efficacy of the newer antiepileptic drugs in controlling seizures in pregnancy. Epilepsia. 2014;55(8):1229–34.
12. Battino D, Tomson T, Bonizzoni E, Craig J, Lindhout D, Sabers A, Perucca E, Vajda F, EURAP Study Group. Seizure control and treatment changes in pregnancy: observations from the EURAP epilepsy pregnancy registry. Epilepsia. 2013;54(9):1621–7.
13. Reisinger TL, Newman M, Loring DW, Pennell PB, Meador KJ. Antiepileptic drug clearance and seizure frequency during pregnancy in women with epilepsy. Epilepsy Behav. 2013;29(1):13–8.
14. Holmes LB, Baldwin EJ, Smith CR, Habecker E, Glassman L, Wong SL, Wyszynski DF. Increased frequency of isolated cleft palate in infants exposed to lamotrigine during pregnancy. Neurology. 2008;70(22 Pt 2):2152–8.
15. Tennis P, Eldridge RR, International Lamotrigine Pregnancy Registry Scientific Advisory Committee. Preliminary results on pregnancy outcomes in women using lamotrigine. Epilepsia. 2002;43:1161–7.

Chapter 7
Seizure Medications and Teratogenicity

David E. Friedman and Torbjörn Tomson

Case Scenario

A 23-year-old woman has medically refractory focal epilepsy with and without secondary generalized tonic-clonic seizures. Her seizures have been controlled in the past 2 years on a combination of topiramate 200 mg twice daily and levetiracetam 1500 mg twice daily. Previous attempts to lower or simplify her medication regimen resulted in seizure recurrence. She has tried oxcarbazepine and lamotrigine in the past with no success. During her visit, she brings up the fact that she desires to become pregnant and start a family. How do you counsel the patient regarding the risks for teratogenicity of her seizure medications and what do you advise her to do?

D.E. Friedman, M.D.
Department of Neuroscience, Winthrop Comprehensive Epilepsy Center,
Winthrop University Hospital, Mineola, NY, USA

Associate Clinical Professor of Neurology, SUNY Stony Brook School of Medicine,
Stony Brook, Mineola, NY 11501, USA
e-mail: defriedman@winthrop.org

T. Tomson, M.D., Ph.D.
Department of Neurology, Karolinska University Hospital,
Karolinska vägen 1, Stockholm 171 76, Sweden
e-mail: torbjorn.tomson@karolinska.se

Commentator: M. Sazgar, M.D. (✉)
University of California, Irvine Medical Center,
101 The City Drive South, Pavilion I, Bldg. 30, Suite 123, Orange, CA 92868, USA
e-mail: msazgar@uci.edu

© Springer International Publishing Switzerland 2016
M. Sazgar, C.L. Harden (eds.), *Controversies in Caring for Women
with Epilepsy*, DOI 10.1007/978-3-319-29170-3_7

Author #1's Response

Introduction

Though most pregnancies among women with epilepsy (WWE) are uneventful, and most babies are delivered healthy with little increased risk of obstetric complications, the management of epilepsy during pregnancy can be challenging for health care providers. There is established and accumulating evidence suggesting an association between prenatal exposure to antiepileptic drugs (AEDs) and increased risk for both physical malformations and neurodevelopmental impairments.

Seizures During Pregnancy

Suboptimal seizure control prior to pregnancy appears to be a reliable predictor of seizure control during pregnancy, and women with monthly seizures are significantly more likely to experience more frequent seizures during pregnancy than those who are seizure-free or have relatively infrequent seizures in the year before conception [1]. One of the major goals in treating all people with epilepsy is to reduce seizures. This is especially relevant during pregnancy, as seizures pose an inherent risk to the health of the fetus in utero. Convulsive seizures represent the strongest risk factor for seizure-related injuries, most often occurring secondary to falls which can lead to fetal trauma. Metabolic abnormalities occur during prolonged convulsive seizures, and fetal hypoxia, bradycardia, decelerations, and death have been reported during tonic-clonic seizures [2]. Fetal decelerations of up to 45 % have been reported during the ictal and immediate postictal phase of complex partial seizures, with effects lasting over 3 min in duration [3, 4], suggesting that non-convulsive seizures may also pose a risk detrimental to the fetus. Because of the serious risk for both maternal and fetal morbidity, the typical recommendation is to continue AED treatment for pregnant WWE.

Potential Teratogenic Effects of AEDs

Though the clinical decision is often to maintain AED therapy during pregnancy, there is a common concern for potential teratogenicity associated with these medications. Early studies warned of the potential dangers of exposure to AEDs in utero, though these were often retrospective. Because of obvious ethical and logistical reasons, no prospective controlled trials have been performed in pregnant WWE. Therefore, the available data from recent pregnancy registries are prospective and observational, and focus primarily on risk for congenital structural anomalies. Though the observational nature of these registries presents methodological

Table 7.1 Risk of major congenital malformations in WWE (%)

	NAAED	UK	Australia	Sweden	Finland	Other
Valproate	10.7	6.2	13.3	9.7	10.7	
Phenobarbital	6.5					
Carbamazepine	2.5	2.2	3.0	4.0	2.7	
Phenytoin			5.9			
Lamotrigine	2.7	3.2	1.4			2.9
Levetiracetam	2.4	2.7				
Topiramate		4.8				9.8

NAAED North American Antiepileptic Drug Pregnancy Registry

limitations, there is increased confidence of results when several independent studies observe similar patterns of drug risk. Because our patient is on topiramate-levetiracetam polytherapy, we should review the available evidence for teratogenic effects specifically associated with these drugs.

Topiramate

Animal studies described an increased risk for craniofacial anomalies in litters exposed to topiramate in utero. Post-marketing studies in pregnant women reported fetal structural malformations associated with topiramate exposure, including cleft lip with or without cleft palate. In 2008, Hunt et al. reported an incidence of cleft lip and cleft palate 11 times the background rate for topiramate-exposed infants in monotherapy [5]. However, this information was based on 2 cases among 70 exposures. Furthermore, the overall rate of all major congenital malformations (MCMs) attributed to topiramate in this report is similar to rates reported in other pregnancy registries for other AEDs (Table 7.1). A recent matched case-control analysis was performed measuring the risk for facial anomalies for children exposed to topiramate in utero, using data from two large congenital malformations case-control studies [6]. Pooled data revealed an increased risk for cleft lip with or without cleft palate compared to children not exposed to AEDs (OR 5.36 [1.49–20.07]). However, risk for developing other major malformations was not observed. Though this study did suggest an increased risk for cleft lip, it too was limited due to a low number of exposed cases.

Levetiracetam

Since 2011, published reports about the risks for fetal malformations described relatively low risk (Table 7.2). Recently, data from the UK and Ireland Epilepsy and Pregnancy Registry reported the risks for anomalies with levetiracetam in

Table 7.2 Major congenital malformations associated with levetiracetam in monotherapy and in polytherapy

	UCB registry	Danish	NAAED	UK and Ireland	Total
Monotherapy	12/253 (4.7 %)	0/58 (0 %)	11/450 (2.4 %)	2/304 (0.66 %)	25/1065 (2.35 %)
Polytherapy	13/105 (12.4 %)			19/367 (5.2 %)	32/472 (6.78 %)

NAAED North American Antiepileptic Drug Pregnancy Registry

monotherapy (304 pregnancies) and polytherapy (367 pregnancies) [7]. There were two cases of major malformations in the monotherapy group (OR 0.7 [0.19–2.51]) and 19 in the polytherapy group (5.56 [3.54–8.56]). With regards to specific AED combinations among those exposed to polytherapy, the rates of malformations were highest with levetiracetam-carbamazepine (9.4 %) and levetiracetam-valproate (6.9 %). No fetal anomalies were reported among the 20 pregnancies exposed to levetiracetam-topiramate.

Potential Cognitive Effects of Fetal Exposure to AEDs

In addition to the increased risk for congenital malformations, fetal exposure to AEDs can lead to cognitive impairment. In recent prospective data, valproate appears to carry the highest risk for future objective cognitive problems [8] and autistic traits [9] when compared to other AEDs. Interestingly, children with fetal exposure to levetiracetam experienced superior language and motor development in comparison to children exposed to valproate when measured at 3–5 years of age [10]. However, there is little information on neurocognitive problems in children exposed to topiramate in utero.

Discussion

Because our patient was at one point refractory, but is now seizure-free, there should be an understandable reluctance in making changes in her regimen, as preconception seizure control is a factor associated with seizures during pregnancy, and seizures during pregnancy carry an inherent risk for the fetus. Previous attempts to make changes in her AED regimen, including dose reduction, led to seizures. Therefore the most conservative approach, strictly taking seizures as a risk for poor outcomes, would be to not make any changes in her medications, as maintaining best seizure control is tantamount to optimizing the health of the fetus. Though there is a risk for potential fetal malformations, the risk is relatively low, though it is recommended that pregnant WWE avoid valproate. Because of the many AEDs used in clinical practice, and the many potential AED combinations, there is a fundamental difficulty in investigating the risks associated with fetal exposure to AED polytherapy. Nevertheless, it is somewhat encouraging for our patient, as there is published data reporting no congenital malformations with topiramate-levetiracetam polytherapy. Recent evidence on neurocognitive outcomes has become available, and levetiracetam was found to be favorable compared to valproate. However, there is no specific data for topiramate.

In providing optimal care and counseling for our patient, we should underscore regular compliance with her medications as well as follow-up visits with her treating neurologists and obstetricians. She should be counseled on the potential obstetric risks, and potential risks to her child, and folate use should be encouraged prior to conception, as some data suggests that initiation later in pregnancy may have little benefit. There should be an emphasis on the fact that most WWE experience uneventful pregnancies and deliver healthy children.

Author #2's Response

Teratogenic Risks with Topiramate and Levetiracetam

Levetiracetam and topiramate belong to the newer generation AEDs, and as such the experience with their use in pregnancy is still limited. This is true regarding their efficacy during pregnancy as well as their potential adverse effects on the fetus in terms of intrauterine growth retardation, risk of congenital malformations, or neurodevelopment. Of the two drugs, levetiracetam is the more studied. Prospective pregnancy registries have reported rates of MCMs ranging from 1 to 2.4 % among children whose mothers were using levetiracetam as monotherapy during pregnancy [11]. However, the number of exposed in each study is still small, 450 in the largest, and the estimates still uncertain. Data on topiramate from the prospective registries are even more scarce, with 359 monotherapy exposures in the largest [11]. Reported MCM rates with topiramate were 2.4–7.7 % [11]. A recent meta-analysis analyzed the risk of one specific MCM, oral clefts, in offspring exposed to topiramate in first trimester [12], and found a sixfold increased risk compared with unexposed, Odds Ratio 6.26 (95 % Confidence Interval 3.13–12.51). So, although data are insufficient for firm conclusions, there are no clear signals of increased MCM risk over other AEDs with levetiracetam, but available data indicate greater risks with topiramate than with, e.g., lamotrigine and carbamazepine.

A population-based nationwide register study from Norway [13] furthermore reports significantly decreased head circumference in newborns of mothers taking topiramate while pregnant, more pronounced than for other AEDs. Whether this effect can have functional consequences for the affected child is unclear. In fact, there are no published systematic prospective studies on the postnatal neurodevelopment of children that have been exposed to topiramate in utero. Information on cognitive outcomes, neurodevelopment, or neurobehavior is also very limited for levetiracetam, comprising one fairly small study assessing development at age 3 [10]. In this study children exposed to levetiracetam scored higher than those exposed to valproate, and not different from unexposed controls [10]. A recent Cochrane review concluded that we have insufficient data on cognitive outcomes about newer AEDs (including levetiracetam and topiramate) [14].

There are two additional concerns related to the teratogenic risks with this young woman's current treatment: (1) The data summarized above are from monotherapy with either of the two drugs; we do not know what risk the specific combination of the two AEDs may carry, although in general polytherapy has been associated with greater fetal risks than monotherapy. (2) No information is available on dose-dependence of the possible teratogenic effects, and we don't know if lower doses than the current might be associated with reduced risks.

In summary is thus clear that our patient's medication is not the ideal for a person planning pregnancy, where the major concern relates to the use of topiramate.

Treatment Options

These risks and uncertainties need to be carefully described and discussed with the patient along with risks and opportunities with relevant treatment alternatives. The ultimate aim with this discussion is to agree on a treatment strategy that is in accordance with the patient's (and partner's) preferences where teratogenic risks as well as risks with possible loss of seizure control need to be considered.

Which are the treatment options in addition to maintaining the current treatment? Fortunately, this patient gives us an opportunity to consider a treatment revision well in advance of pregnancy. Never the less, any change of the treatment is associated with a risk regarding seizure control. This is something that has to be explained to and, if attempted, be acceptable for the patient. One option, although maybe less realistic, would be to try gradual withdrawal of both AEDs aiming at no medication at the time of conception. Another option could be to aim at monotherapy with levetiracetam, thereby eliminating the possible teratogenic effects of topiramate, which are likely to be more relevant than those of levetiracetam. A further option would be to try to switch from topiramate to another AED, hopefully with less teratogenic potential but still effective in controlling the patient's seizures. However, as our woman has failed on lamotrigine and oxcarbazepine, the only untried AED with documented favorable teratogenic profile is carbamazepine.

We need more information on this case in order to help our patient with a balanced risk–benefit analysis of the various treatment options, in particular concerning risks of seizure recurrence with AED modifications. She has been considered to have "medically refractory epilepsy" but we really don't know details of her history other than that she failed on two AEDs. Did it take several years before she was rendered seizure free, and do we know anything about the etiology of her epilepsy? A long delay in obtaining remission, and an underlying structural etiology, suggests that the risk of recurrence is high on medication withdrawal, and speak against attempts to withdraw both AEDs. On the other hand, with these factors absent, there could be a chance of successful tapering of topiramate after 2 years seizure freedom. In fact we don't know if she became seizure free after adding levetiracetam to topiramate or vice versa.

A more cautious approach, though not without risk of recurrence would be to keep levetiracetam but try to switch topiramate to carbamazepine as add-on. Regardless of which treatment approach is selected, it needs to be a shared decision based on the preference of the fully informed woman with epilepsy. And when the decision has been made, it is the physician's duty to support the patient and to try to reduce the risks be they teratogenic or associated with seizure recurrence.

Reviewer's Comments

The potential for teratogenic side effects of seizure medications is an ongoing challenge for WWE of childbearing age and for their treating physicians. The first author points out the importance of seizure freedom during pregnancy and the reported risks to the fetus from maternal seizures including but not limited to trauma from maternal falls, fetal hypoxia, heart rate decelerations, and death. He leans toward keeping the patient stable on her anticonvulsant medications. Teramo and colleagues studied three WWE who experienced generalized tonic-clonic seizure during labor [15]. There were marked changes in fetal heart rate for up to 60 min after the seizure. There was also a risk for increased uterine contractions during and after a seizure, resulting in decreased arterial blood flow to the placenta. To avoid the potential harmful effects of convulsive or prolonged partial seizures on the fetus and expectant mother, the general practice is to keep a patient with epilepsy on anticonvulsant therapy during a pregnancy. This makes "gradual withdrawal of both of patients' seizure medications prior to pregnancy" which is listed by the second author as an option, to be less favorable.

The other option discussed by Author #2 is an attempt with monotherapy on levetiracetam. However previous attempts in changing either of her medications in this patient have resulted in seizure recurrence. This option will work if the patient belongs to the subgroup of WWE who have improvement in their seizures during pregnancy. The first author acknowledges that although not ideal to keep the patient on both medications, it may well be our most practical option. This is based on the only limited piece of data obtained from the UK and Ireland Epilepsy and Pregnancy Registry which reported no fetal anomalies among the 20 pregnancies exposed to levetiracetam-topiramate polytherapy. This number is not sufficient to make firm conclusions regarding the safety of this combination. Topiramate in the United States is moved to pregnancy category D based on positive evidence of human fetal risks mentioned by both authors.

Suggested Management

1. In WWE considering pregnancy, all attempts must be made to simplify seizure medication regimen and if possible achieve monotherapy.
2. The pregnancy registries data on levetiracetam so far is favorable and show no significant risk for MCM.
3. Topiramate is pregnancy category D in the United States due to significantly increasing the risk for oral clefts and should be avoided in women considering pregnancy unless there is no other choice and the benefits outweigh the risks.

References

1. Tanganelli P, Regesta G. Epilepsy, pregnancy, and major birth anomalies: an Italian prospective, controlled study. Neurology. 1992;42(4 Suppl 5):89–93.
2. Hiilemsa VK, Teramo K, Bardy AH. Social class, complications, and perinatal deaths in pregnancies of epileptic women: preliminary results of the prospective Helsinki study. In: Janz D, editor. Epilepsy, pregnancy, and the child. New York: Raven; 1982. p. 53–9.
3. Nei M, Daly S, Liporace J. A maternal complex partial seizure in labor can affect fetal heart rate. Neurology. 1998;51(3):904–6.
4. Sahoo S, Klein P. Maternal complex partial seizure associated with fetal distress. Arch Neurol. 2005;62(8):1304–5.
5. Hunt S, Russell A, Smithson WH, et al. Topiramate in pregnancy: preliminary experience from the UK Epilepsy and Pregnancy Register. Neurology. 2008;71(4):272–6.
6. Margulis AV, Mitchell AA, Gilboa SM, et al. Use of topiramate in pregnancy and risk of oral clefts. Am J Obstet Gynecol. 2012;207(5):405e1–7.
7. Mawhinney E, Craig J, Morrow J, et al. Levetiracetam in pregnancy: results from the UK and Ireland epilepsy and pregnancy registers. Neurology. 2013;80(4):400–5.
8. Meador KJ, Baker GA, Browning N, et al. Cognitive function at 3 years of age after fetal exposure to antiepileptic drugs. N Engl J Med. 2009;360(16):1597–605.
9. Wood AG, Nadebaum C, Anderson V, et al. Prospective assessment of autism traits in children exposed to antiepileptic drugs during pregnancy. Epilepsia. 2015;56(7):1047–55.
10. Shallcorss R, Bromley RL, Cheyne CP, et al. In utero exposure to levetiracetam versus valproate: development and language at 3 years of age. Neurology. 2014;82(3):213–21.
11. Tomson T, Xue H, Battino D. Major congenital malformations in children of women with epilepsy. Seizure. 2015;28:46–50. http://dx.doi.org/10.1016/j.seizure.2015.02.019.
12. Veiby G, Daltveit AK, Engelsen BA, et al. Fetal growth restriction and birth defects with newer and older antiepileptic drugs during pregnancy. J Neurol. 2014;261(3):579–88.
13. Bromley R, Weston J, Adab N, et al. Treatment for epilepsy in pregnancy: neurodevelopmental outcomes in the child. Cochrane Database Syst Rev. 2014;10:CD010236. doi:10.1002/14651858. CD010236.pub2.
14. Alsaad AMS, Chaudhry SA, Koren G. First trimester exposure to topiramate and the risk of oral clefts in the offspring: a systematic review and meta-analysis. Reprod Toxicol. 2015;53:45–50. http://dx.doi.org/10.1016/j.reprotox.2015.03.003.
15. Teramo K, Hiilesmaa V, Bardy A, Saarikoski S. Fetal heart rate during a maternal grand mal epileptic seizure. J Perinat Med. 1979;7:3–6.

Chapter 8
Valproic Acid and Pregnancy: Failed Other Medications

Fábio A. Nascimento, Lara V. Marcuse, and Danielle M. Andrade

Case Scenario

A 25-year-old woman was diagnosed with Juvenile Myoclonic Epilepsy (JME) since age 13. She was tried on lamotrigine which resulted in full body rash. She has failed other medications including topiramate, zonisamide, and levetiracetam due to lack of efficacy for controlling her seizures. She has been managed with valproic acid in the past 5 years with no reported seizure recurrence. She would like to get pregnant in the next year or two. How would you counsel her and what treatment changes would you make, if any?

F.A. Nascimento, M.D.
Division of Neurology, Toronto Western Hospital, University of Toronto,
5W-445, 399, Bathurst St., Toronto, ON, Canada M5T 2S8
e-mail: Nascimento.Fabio.A@gmail.com

L.V. Marcuse, M.D.
Department of Neurology, Mount Sinai, 1 Gustave Levy Place, New York, NY 11226, USA
e-mail: lara.marcuse@mountsinai.org

D.M. Andrade, M.D., M.Sc.
Medical Director, Epilepsy Program, Krembil Neuroscience, Director of Epilepsy Genetics
Research Program, Director, Epilepsy Transition Program, Associate Professor,
Neurology, University of Toronto, Toronto, ON, Canada M5T 2S8
e-mail: danielle.andrade@uhn.ca

Commentator: C.L. Harden, M.D. (✉)
Mount Sinai Health System, Mount Sinai Beth Israel Phillips Ambulatory Care Center,
10 Union Square East, Suite 5D, New York, NY 10003, USA
e-mail: charden@chpnet.org

© Springer International Publishing Switzerland 2016
M. Sazgar, C.L. Harden (eds.), *Controversies in Caring for Women
with Epilepsy*, DOI 10.1007/978-3-319-29170-3_8

AUTHOR #1'S RESPONSE

*Epilepsy is a disease of a peculiarly serious and revolting character, tending to weaken mental force, and often descending from parent to child, or entailing upon the offspring of the sufferer some other grave form of nervous malady.—*Gould v. Gould, 78 Conn. 246, 61 Atl. 604 (1905)

At the turn of the century in this country, eugenics laws in many states made it illegal for people with epilepsy to marry and in some cases there was forced steriliza-tion. As twenty-first century epileptologists seeking to empower (and not oppress) our patients, it may be time to shed the cloak of paternalism, particularly as there is often no clear answer. Perhaps we should see ourselves as a guide, digesting the complex web of data and presenting it in as clear a manner as possible so that each woman can have support and information for making the decisions that are best for her.

The Risk to the Baby

Prospective pregnancy registries have condemned valproic acid as the most terato-genic antiepileptic drug (AED) on the market today. In the North American preg-nancy registry, the rate of major malformations with valproic acid monotherapy was 9.3 %. This compares poorly to rates of major malformations of 2 %, 2.4 %, and 4.2 % for lamotrigine, levetiracetam, and topiramate, respectively. In this regis-try zonegran had 0 malformations but there were only 90 offspring evaluated, result-ing in wide confidence intervals [1].

The European registry of antiepileptic drugs and pregnancy (EURAP) provides more nuanced data regarding the dose-dependent risk of AEDs in pregnancy. For all four AEDs reported (valproic acid, phenobarbital, carbamazepine, and lamotrig-ine), there was an increase in major malformations with increasing dose (Fig. 8.1). Specifically for valproic acid the major malformation rate was 4.2 % at a dose less than 700 mg, 9.0 at a dose between 700 and 1500 mg, and a very unfortunate 23 % for a dose of greater than 1500 mg [2].

Furthermore, the risk of valproic acid has a farther reach than major malformations. The neurodevelopmental effects of anti-epileptic drug (NEAD) study group examined the cognitive outcome of children exposed to valproic acid, phenytoin, lamotrigine, or carbamazepine in monotherapy. Valproic acid was associated with lower IQ at all age points tested. At 6 years, the adjusted mean IQ for children in the valproic acid group was 97, 7–10 points lower than the IQ of children on the other medications tested [3].

For valproic acid, all of the neurodevelopmental outcomes had a dose response relationship with less of an impact for the lower doses of valproic acid [3]. Higher doses of valproic acid were associated with diminished non-verbal and verbal skills as well as reduced executive function and memory. Importantly for our patient, at doses of <1000 mg of valproic acid the cognitive outcomes did not differ between the chil-dren exposed to valproic acid compared to children exposed to the other AEDs [3].

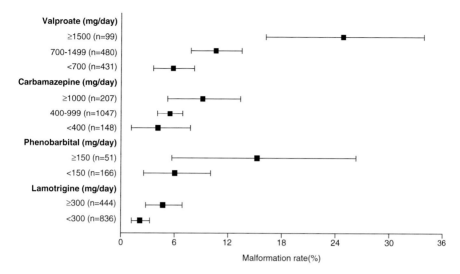

Fig. 8.1 Rates of major congenital malformations at 1 year after birth in relation to exposure to antiepileptic drug monotherapy. *Bars* are 95 % CI (From Tomson T, Battino D. Teratogenic effects of antiepileptic drugs. Lancet Neurol 2012; 11: 803–13 with permission)

Seizures and the Risk to the Mother

Most epileptologists have patients with idiopathic generalized epilepsy who are difficult to control on any medication except for valproic acid. Head-to-head efficacy trials in epilepsy are few and far between, but there is one trial confirming our experience in the clinic and that is the SANAD trial [4]. In this trial, patients with idiopathic generalized or unclassified epilepsy (both genders and not pregnant) were randomized to receive valproic acid, topiramate, or lamotrigine. Valproic acid was superior in terms of seizure control to both other medications in the patients with idiopathic generalized epilepsy [4].

Higher doses of AEDs seem to be associated with worsened seizure control for women on any of the four medications analyzed (carbamazepine, lamotrigine, phenobarbital, and valproic acid) [5]. Women taking valproic acid at its least teratogenic dose of <700 mg experienced seizures in 22.2 % of pregnancies. Women taking valproic acid at its most teratogenic dose of >1500 mg had seizures in 32.3 % of pregnancies [5]. The increased seizure frequency in women taking the higher dose is surely secondary to the more difficult nature of their epilepsy. Yet, these numbers are somewhat re-assuring and suggest that a lower dose of <700 mg of valproic acid per day may be effective for many women.

In considering safety and seizures for our 25-year-old woman with idiopathic generalized epilepsy, the details of her epilepsy are important. Five years of seizure freedom is always a good prognostic sign and indicates the possibility that she could reduce the dose of valproic acid or even consider changing to a previously known-to-be-less efficacious medication like levetiracetam. If her history on the other medications is one of frequent and uncontrolled generalized tonic-clonic convulsions, then this avenue is very unappealing. If her seizures were poorly controlled in adolescence in part due to poor sleep and a tendency to binge drink at parties, it is conceivable that a return to another broad-spectrum AED with the added antiepileptic treatment of self-care could be effective.

If she lives in Brooklyn and never drives a vehicle, this may give her more flexibility in trying a different treatment plan with an increased risk of seizures than if she works as a truck driver traversing the country with all night driving.

Seizures and the Risk to the Baby

Interestingly, seizure freedom during pregnancy did not decrease the risk of malformations. In fact, the relationship appears somewhat inversed (Fig. 8.2). When lamotrigine, phenobarbital, carbamazepine, and valproic acid are compared, patients on lamotrigine (least teratogenic) have the highest risk of seizures and patients taking valproic acid (most teratogenic) have the lowest risk of seizures [1].

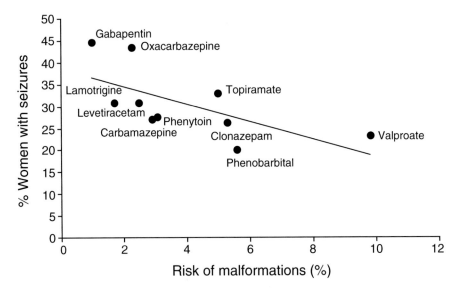

Fig. 8.2 Risk of major malformations by proportion of women having at least one seizure during their pregnancy within each antiepileptic drug group among women with epilepsy. North American AED Pregnancy Registry 1997–2011 (From Hernandez-Díaz S, Smith CR, Shen A, Mittendorf R, Hauser, WA, Yerby M, Holmes, LB; North American AED Pregnancy Registry. Comparative safety of antiepileptic drugs during pregnancy. Neurology 2012; 78: 1692–9. doi: 10.1212/WNL.0b013e3182574f39. Epub 2012 May 2 with permission)

However, this line of thinking should not be pursued with abandon as in the 21 cases of status epilepticus reported in the EURAP registry, there were three major malformations, representing a risk of 14 % and suggesting that uncontrolled seizure could contribute to major malformations [5].

Having the Conversation

There is no clear right avenue for our 25-year-old women. The best approach is to outline what is known about pregnancy and epilepsy clearly and simply and to review the nuances and data of her history. Then a plan can be generated jointly by the doctor and the patient.

The basic principles of pregnancy and epilepsy should be adhered to. Unplanned pregnancy occurs in all cultures throughout the world and in all socioeconomic classes. It is our job to review and actively discuss the safety of a woman's regime regarding pregnancy even when she is not trying to get pregnant. Supplementation with folic acid is reasonable. With idiopathic generalized epilepsy, self-care with good sleep and a regular schedule can be very helpful.

Preplanning is best! A year or two jumpstart in pregnancy to get the most sensical treatment is optimal. Based on the evidence and depending on her specific history, the primary discussion points would be to either lower the dose of valproic acid (<700 mg) or to change to a broad-spectrum medication that is less teratogenic.

AUTHOR #2'S RESPONSE

The Valproate in Pregnancy Dilemma: Is There a Safe Prescription?

Peri-conception counselling and care remain the most efficacious strategy to improve the chances of a favorable pregnancy outcome. Generally, more than 90 % of women with epilepsy have a completely normal pregnancy. With proper instructions and management during the perigestational period, this figure can still be increased. In other words, this whole process of care is of paramount importance and usually translated into a healthy mother–baby binomial. From now onward, we shall focus on the patient presented in the *case scenario* above.

Our patient is a 25-year-old lady, hypothetically named Kathy Smith (KS), who was diagnosed with JME at the age of 13. She has been tried on several AEDs, including lamotrigine, levetiracetam, topiramate, and zonisamide. All of them, either due to side effect or failure to control seizures, were discontinued. Valproate, however, was well tolerated and has made her seizure-free for the past 5 years. No real challenge up to this point. Nonetheless, clinical picture changes completely when she states the desire to start a family in the next couple of years. Despite the fact that this scenario is fairly common, many controversies still permeate this particular clinical situation. Let us begin the discussion with a brief overview of JME.

JME, a genetic epilepsy syndrome, typically occurs in otherwise healthy adolescents and is classically characterized by the triad of myoclonic jerks, generalized tonic-clonic seizures, and absence seizures. These epileptic events happen generally upon awakening; as of triggers, the most significant of them is sleep deprivation. JME patients respond quite well and rapidly to broad-spectrum AED therapy. The first-line drug is valproate, which has a response rate of up to 80 %. Levetiracetam or lamotrigine are alternative first choice options if valproate is for some reason contraindicated. Concerning prognosis, seizure frequency often is reduced in adulthood (mainly by the fourth decade of life) but most patients require lifelong antiepileptic treatment.

Women with epilepsy, regardless of the specific epileptic syndrome, are at increased risk of a number of potential obstetrical and fetal complications. These complications, which essentially derive from maternal seizures and epilepsy, as well as from effects of AEDs on the fetus, can be divided into three categories: obstetrical complications, perinatal mortality and miscarriage, and fetal maldevelopment due to antiepileptic treatment. Given that these complications are secondary to occurrence of seizures and/or teratogenic effects of antiepileptic treatment, the goal of management is clear: to achieve seizure control/freedom with the most appropriate (less teratogenic) AED at the lowest dose possible.

The first reasonable idea that comes to mind when facing KS in clinic is to try her off anticonvulsant treatment and evaluate her response. However, as previously mentioned, JME patients usually require chronic and sustained antiepileptic therapy. Most of these individuals, if discontinuation of AED(s) is tried, relapse—fact that can be explained by the lifelong character of JME. Recurrence of seizures would be too risky, especially in the setting of an ongoing pregnancy. Hence, weaning KS off medication is not a good option. The second idea would be to switch her from valproate to another AED. It would not be, however, doable—due to the fact that she has failed alternative AEDs that traditionally work well on controlling JME. Therefore, we finally reach the real clinical challenge: to control her seizures at the perigestational period utilizing valproate, one of the most teratogenic anticonvulsants.

Classified as a category D drug by the Food and Drug Administration (FDA), valproate and its products "should be used in pregnant women with epilepsy only if other treatments have failed to provide adequate symptom control or are otherwise unacceptable." In the context of pregnancy, the adverse effects of VPA essentially relate to three domains: fetal malformations (FMs), long-term cognitive effects, and higher chances of autism spectrum disorders (ASD). Congenital malformations include neural tube defects, cardiovascular and urogenital abnormalities, craniofacial anomalies, and musculoskeletal defects. In terms of cognitive effects, recent well-designed prospective studies showed that children exposed to high doses of VPA in utero had lower IQ scores at age of 6 years compared to kids not exposed to any AED, those exposed to low doses of VPA, and those exposed to other AED(s) [3, 6]. Regarding ASD, a major population-based study from Denmark concluded that VPA use during pregnancy was associated with significantly increased risk of ASD [7].

Interestingly, it has been established that VPA's teratogenicity is dose-related. Higher total daily doses of VPA (especially in the first trimester of pregnancy) are associated with higher risks of fetal malformations as well as with long-term learning problems and lower cognitive performance—but not with the higher chances of developing ASD. The risk of adverse congenital structural and functional effects increases significantly at total daily doses of 700 mg and above. Daily doses lower than this figure are associated with an FM rate in a similar range as that of other select AEDs (lamotrigine, phenobarbital, and carbamazepine) [8]. On the same note, spina bifida and hypospadias appear to be the types of malformations that bear the most important quantitative relationship to drug dose [9]. Regarding cognitive outcome, the deleterious effect is present in kids who were exposed in utero to doses of VPA over 800 mg per day. Children exposed to less than 800 mg per day of VPA, on the other hand, were assessed to have normal cognition and IQ scores [6].

After *sorting through the evidence*, we would initially reassure KS that the majority of women with epilepsy have a normal pregnancy and healthy babies. Subsequently, we would reinforce the importance of avoiding seizure triggers (especially sleep deprivation, in patients with JME), and of having a healthy lifestyle. As to AED therapy, we would lower her total daily dose of valproate to less than 700 mg. Concomitantly, we would supplement her with 4 mg of folic acid per day, once her baby is at risk of neural tube defects.

There would be two possible outcomes on decreasing her AED: (1) continued seizure control, or (2) seizure recurrence. In response to the first, we would maintain the same strategy, trying to settle the valproate at the lowest effective dosage. In case low doses of valproate fail to control her epilepsy, outcome (2), we would add a second AED—a benzodiazepine (BZD), such as clonazepam or clobazam. The rationale for electing a BZD as the additional anticonvulsant, in this particular context, resides mainly in the minimal teratogenic potential of BZDs. Although some case-control studies did suggest a twofold increase in the risk of oral cleft, several cohort studies failed to show any association between fetal exposure to BZD and birth defects [10, 11]. Lastly, in the event that we do add a BZD to her AED regimen, we would involve a neonatologist in her perinatal care, since BZD use (especially close to delivery) can cause neonatal toxicity and withdrawal. Acute toxic effects on neonates include hypotonia, hypoglycemia, poor feeding, and respiratory depression. Neonatal withdrawal, which typically presents hours to weeks after birth and may persist for a few months, consists of irritability, hyperactivity, hyperreflexia, hyper- or hypotonia, tremors, vomiting, among others [12].

In conclusion, in order to maximize the chances of a healthy pregnancy, clinicians should always try to control patients' seizures with the less teratogenic AED at the lowest effective dose. Importantly, this goal should be achieved, ideally, prior to conception; therefore the major importance of active counselling about planning pregnancy. Fortunately, with proper, early, and careful management the vast majority of pregnancies will have successful outcomes.

Reviewer's Comments

The authors reviewing this difficult case both arrived at the same conclusion, which is that the evidence supports continuing valproate at a dose of 700 mg per day or less. Author #2 offered a further management approach, should seizures occur, which is to add a low dose benzodiazepine. The risks to the fetal development, as poorly known as they are, and the risks to the neonate at delivery were presented, along with management approaches for a sedated, potentially low-tone newborn. This author also discussed JME in general, serving to underscore the ongoing seizure risk associated with the syndrome, even when seizures are well-controlled. This is important because JME and its treatment will affect this patient for future pregnancies and future life epochs.

Author #1 presents the provocative evidence that seizures during pregnancy, from one of the largest observational studies available, were not associated with increased risk of major malformations. The drug exposure was of course, with valproate associating with the greatest risk, followed by phenobarbital, clonazepam, and topiramate. This makes the joint decision-making complex in this case. Women may want to go the route of risking seizures to protect their pregnancy, while health care providers are focused on the safety and well-being of patient in front of them, and are acutely aware of the dangers of letting seizures happen.

One of these dangers is sudden unexpected death in epilepsy (SUDEP). A recent, population-based study from the United Kingdom Confidential Enquiry into Maternal Death Registry from 2006 to 2008 captured deaths in women with epilepsy while pregnant including up to 42 days after termination of pregnancy [13]. The SUDEP incidence rate was 0.79 per 1000 pregnancies (95 % CI 0.6–1.0), which is approximately twice as high as other studies using the general population of persons with epilepsy [14, 15]. Women with epilepsy are at risk for this most dire complication of epilepsy, and this is one of the many important reasons for caregivers promoting seizure control during pregnancy.

Suggested Management

1. Valproate at less than or equal to 700 mg per day for women who have not responded to other antiseizure medications and are well-controlled presents a favorable risk to benefit balance for continuing this dose during pregnancy.
2. Seizure occurrence during pregnancy is not correlated with increased rate of major congenital malformations. However, seizures are known to result in trauma, falls, fetal hypoxia, fetal heart rate deceleration, and other potential harmful effects.
3. The option of adding a benzodiazepine for seizure control may be considered if low dose valproate fails to control seizures during pregnancy. In that case, one should watch for signs of neonatal benzodiazepine withdrawal for days or weeks after delivery.

References

1. Hernandez-Díaz S, Smith CR, Shen A, Mittendorf R, Hauser WA, Yerby M, Holmes LB, North American AED Pregnancy Registry. Comparative safety of antiepileptic drugs during pregnancy. Neurology. 2012;78:1692–9. doi:10.1212/WNL.0b013e3182574f39. Epub 2012 May 2.
2. Tomson T, Battino D. Teratogenic effects of antiepileptic drugs. Lancet Neurol. 2012;11:803–13.
3. Meador KJ, Baker GA, Browning N, Cohen MJ, Bromley RL, Clayton-Smith J, Kalayjian LA, Kanner A, Liporace JD, Pennell PB, Privitera M, Loring DW, NEAD Study Group. Fetal antiepileptic drug exposure and cognitive outcomes at age 6 years (NEAD study): a prospective observational study. Lancet Neurol. 2013;12(3):244–52.
4. Marson AG, Al-Kharusi AM, Alwaidh M, Appleton R, Baker GA, Chadwick DW, et al, SANAD Study group. The SANAD study of effectiveness of valproate, lamotrigine, or topiramate for generalised and unclassifiable epilepsy: an unblinded randomised controlled trial. Lancet. 2007;369(9566):1016–26.
5. Battino D, Tomson T, Bonizzoni E, Craig J, Lindhout D, Sabers A, Perucca E, Vajda F, EURAP Study Group. Seizure control and treatment changes in pregnancy: observations from the EURAP epilepsy pregnancy registry. Epilepsia. 2013;54(9):1621–7.
6. Baker GA, Bromley RL, Briggs M, Cheyne CP, Cohen MJ, Garcia-Finana M, et al, Liverpool and Manchester Neurodevelopment Group. IQ at 6 years after in utero exposure to antiepileptic drugs: a controlled cohort study. Neurology. 2015;84(4):382–90.
7. Christensen J, Gronborg TK, Sorensen MJ, Schendel D, Parner ET, Pedersen LH, Vestergaard M. Prenatal valproate exposure and risk of autism spectrum disorders and childhood autism. JAMA. 2013;309(16):1696–703.
8. Tomson T, Battino D. Teratogenic effects of antiepileptic drugs. Lancet Neurol. 2012;11(9):803–13.
9. Vajda FJ, O'Brien TJ, Graham JE, Lander CM, Eadie MJ. Dose dependence of fetal malformations associated with valproate. Neurology. 2013;81(11):999–1003.
10. Dolovich LR, Addis A, Vaillancourt JM, Power JD, Koren G, Einarson TR. Benzodiazepine use in pregnancy and major malformations or oral cleft: meta-analysis of cohort and case-control studies. BMJ. 1998;317(7162):839–43.
11. Enato E, Moretti M, Koren G. The fetal safety of benzodiazepines: an updated meta-analysis. J Obstet Gynaecol Can. 2011;33(1):46–8.
12. Hudak ML, Tan RC, Committee on Drugs, Committee on Fetus and Newborn, American Academy of Pediatrics. Neonatal drug withdrawal. Pediatrics. 2012;129(2):e540–60.
13. Edey S, Moran N, Nashef L. SUDEP and epilepsy-related mortality in pregnancy. Epilepsia. 2014;55(7):e72–4.
14. Tennis P, Cole TB, Annegers JF, Leestma JE, McNutt M, Rajput A. Cohort study of incidence of sudden unexplained death in persons with seizure disorder treated with antiepileptic drugs in Saskatchewan, Canada. Epilepsia. 1995;1:29–36.
15. Aurlien D, Larsen JP, Gjerstad L, Taubøll E. Comorbid and underlying diseases—major determinants of excess mortality in epilepsy. Seizure. 2012;21(8):573–7.

Chapter 9
Valproic Acid and Pregnancy: Not Tried Other Medications

Nigar Dargah-zada, Cynthia L. Harden, and Anne Sabers

Case Scenario

A 24-year-old woman was diagnosed with juvenile myoclonic epilepsy (JME) since age 14 and managed by her pediatric neurologist. She has been successfully treated and remained seizure free on valproic acid 500 mg twice daily for several years. She has never been tried on any other seizure medications. She has a full-time job as a real estate agent and drives clients around the city. She reports no side effects on valproic acid. She has been transferred to your care as an adult neurologist. She got married 2 years ago and is planning to become pregnant and start a family in the next year or two. How would you counsel her regarding the risks for teratogenicity of her seizure medication and what treatment changes would you make, if any?

N. Dargah-zada, M.D.
Department of Neurology, Mount Sinai Beth Israel,
E. 16th and 1st Avenue, New York, NY 10003, USA
e-mail: nzada@chpnet.org

C.L. Harden, M.D.
Mount Sinai Health System, Mount Sinai Beth Israel Phillips Ambulatory Care Center,
10 Union Square East, Suite 5D, New York, NY 10003, USA
e-mail: charden@chpnet.org

A. Sabers, M.D., D.M.Sc.
Department of Neurology, Rigshospitalet, Blegdamsvej 9, Copenhagen 2000, Denmark
e-mail: anne.sabers@regionh.dk

Commentator: M. Sazgar, M.D. (✉)
University of California, Irvine Medical Center,
101 The City Drive South, Pavilion I, Bldg. 30, Suite 123, Orange, CA 92868, USA
e-mail: msazgar@uci.edu

© Springer International Publishing Switzerland 2016   73
M. Sazgar, C.L. Harden (eds.), *Controversies in Caring for Women with Epilepsy*, DOI 10.1007/978-3-319-29170-3_9

AUTHOR #1'S RESPONSE

JME is best controlled with valproic acid, being treatment of choice as monotherapy, since 80 % of patients can be seizure free on valproic acid therapy [1]. However in certain circumstances, such as the occurrence of side effects, inadequate seizure control, and most importantly for the case under discussion, teratogenic risks during pregnancy [2], other treatment options should be considered. Since monotherapy is associated with less teratogenic risk than polytherapy [3], monotherapy alternatives to valproic acid for JME will be discussed. Four antiseizure medications are reasonable to consider: these are levetiracetam, lamotrigine, topiramate, and zonisamide. Lamotrigine, levetiracetam, zonisamide, and topiramate have shown to have similar efficacy to valproic acid (VPA) for controlling JME seizures; however, each has its special concerns.

Levetiracetam may be used as primary agent in the treatment of JME [4]. This medication has a good safety profile, has proven efficacy, and can be initiated readily at a known therapeutic dose. Levetiracetam monotherapy may reduce seizure frequency by up to 60 % in patients with intractable JME [5]. Both myoclonic seizures and generalized tonic-clonic seizures in patients with JME have been highly responsive to the treatment with levetiracetam. Available information also indicates a low risk of teratogenicity of approximately 2 % [2]. Therefore, levetiracetam should be considered as either the primary or, an adjunct therapy in pregnant patient with JME.

Lamotrigine use is somewhat nuanced; it provides good control of generalized tonic-clonic seizures; however, it may also exacerbate myoclonic jerks, which is of concern in patients presenting primarily with myoclonic jerks component [5, 6]. To avoid lamotrigine's myoclonic effect, clonazepam may be used as adjunct. However this polytherapy regimen is not necessarily optimal in pregnant patients, given exposure to one more medication, which may have potential teratogenic effects and/or risk for neonatal benzodiazepine withdrawal "floppy infant syndrome" symptoms, especially when used in third trimester of pregnancy [7]. The teratogenic risk for lamotrigine is overall low, at approximately 2 % [2].

Topiramate can also be considered the alternative to valproic acid as medication of choice, since it has shown to be effective in controlling 50 % of generalized tonic-clonic seizures as an add-on in the patients with JME in two multicenter, double-blind, randomized, placebo-controlled, parallel-group trials [8]. However, topiramate has been associated with increased risk of cleft lip/palate when used in the first trimester of pregnancy [9] and has a teratogenic rate of approximately 4 % [2]; therefore it is not an absolutely safe option. Nevertheless when compared to the risk of teratogenicity with valproic acid, this medication should still be considered, if seizures are well controlled on it prior to pregnancy.

Zonisamide is generally well tolerated and effective in patients with JME (80 % of patients in one study of 15 subjects showed good control of their seizures on

ZNS monotherapy), but more data is needed to determine its use as monotherapy in patients with JME [10]. Since our patient is a well-educated patient, in this case it is reasonable to go over the studies performed with these drugs to discuss the most preferable plan of therapy for the patient.

Valproic acid certainly remains the treatment of choice for patients with JME, due to its highest efficacy in seizure control. However, extensive teratogenic potential of this medication, used either as mono- or polytherapy, including significant neural tube developmental defects, facial clefts, cardiac defects, hypospadias, and also increased risk of poor cognitive outcomes in babies, exposed to VPA in utero, makes this drug unfavorable in the treatment of pregnant patients.

The risk of major congenital malformations (MCMs) is higher than with the other AEDs discussed here with a rate of 9 % when taken during the first trimester of pregnancy as monotherapy [2]. Also AED polytherapy in the first trimester that included VPA has been shown to contribute to higher risk of MCMs development, when compared to other polytherapy regimens that did not include VPA during the first trimester [3]. Most recent study of the EURAP group has shown that teratogenic effect of valproic acid is, however, strongly correlating to its dosage, and in the smaller doses, the teratogenic potential significantly decreases. The study has shown that the frequency of MCMs is associated with high VPA doses, with the most MCMs occurring at doses >1500 mg. The study has also shown that dose <700 mg/day is associated with decreased frequencies of MCMs. This MCM risk was unchanged both in the presence and absence of a concomitant therapy. The North American AED pregnancy registry has reported the lowest MCMs occurrence at dosages less than 500 mg/day; therefore, it is reasonable to consider lowest doses possible for the use in patients on valproic acid therapy who are planning to conceive [11].

For our patient, there are several different approaches that should be discussed. First of all, since the patient has addressed issue of treatment modification early enough prior to the planned pregnancy, it is reasonable to go over all the options available for treatment of the JME, alternative to VPA therapy, since some of the medications may seem more attractive in light of lighter teratogenic potential. It is worth attempting to switch medications regimen, especially since she has not been tried on medications, other than valproic acid, and response may be surprisingly positive. If the alternative treatment options fail to control seizures adequately, it is reasonable to try to decrease the valproic acid dose from 1000 mg/day, that was efficacious for this patient, to smaller dose, preferably <700 mg/day, and if this fails to control the seizures, it can be advised to use Levetiracetam as adjunct medication, in an attempt to keep valproic acid dosage as low as possible, along with controlling seizures adequately. Patient should also be advised, that general lifestyle modifications should be followed, such as sleep pattern disturbances, psychosocial stress, and alcohol consumption avoidance, and she should be followed closely throughout her pregnancy with the neurologist, who should also be able to provide her with recommendations on epilepsy management after the delivery of her child.

AUTHOR #2'S RESPONSE

General Considerations

In approaching this case, it is mandatory first of all to verify the diagnosis and evaluate the need for continued prophylactic antiepileptic treatment. In general, exposure to antiepileptic drugs during pregnancy increases the risk of congenital major malformations from the background risk of 1–2 to 4–9 %. When this woman has been seizure-free for several years the epilepsy might be in remission. JME, however, is generally regarded as a lifelong condition that tends to recur after withdrawal of antiepileptic medication even after many years of seizure freedom which means that in case her epilepsy syndrome has been correctly classified, she most likely will need continued antiepileptic medication throughout a coming pregnancy.

Given this putative need for continued antiepileptic drug treatment, the essentials in appropriate pre-pregnancy counseling will be to provide her with information that enables her to make informed and shared decisions, assisted by the clinician. The counseling should in particular address the potential teratogenic risks associated with continued treatment with valproic acid versus another antiepileptic drug and balanced against the potential risks associated with seizure recurrence in addition to a potential delay in regaining seizure control in case of changing the medication.

Teratogenic Risk Associated with Valproic Acid vs. Other Antiepileptic Drugs

Several large prospective registry-based studies have confirmed that maternal treatment with valproic acid during pregnancy in general carries greater risk for somatic birth defects in the offspring compared to most other antiepileptic drugs. Additional evidence also link maternal use of valproic acid during pregnancy to neurodevelopmental deficits manifested by cognitive impairments [12] and autistic spectrum disorders in the offspring. Based on these overall observations the European Medicines Agency has recently strengthened warnings on the use of valproic acid for women of childbearing potential in general unless alternative treatments are ineffective or not tolerated.

When considering changing the antiepileptic drug the most obvious antiepileptic alternatives to valproic acid for JME are lamotrigine or levetiracetam. Studies have demonstrated that the rate of major structural malformation is significantly and at least threefold higher for valproic acid monotherapy (ranges from 6.2 to 9.7 %) compared to lamotrigine [13]. The teratogenic risk of levetiracetam is only studied in relative minor studies but is generally also regarded as having a lower teratogenic potential compared to valproic acid.

There is, however, also growing and relative strong evidence that the total daily dose of valproic acid is an important factor for the risk of teratogenicity including the neurodevelopmental disorders. The malformation rate associated with exposure of antiepileptic drugs increases dose-dependently and use of lower doses of valproic acid does not necessarily mean higher risk for cognitive malformations than what is related to use of higher doses of other drugs. In consistency with other studies, the large EURAP study demonstrated that valproic acid in doses of less than 700 mg per day were not associated with higher MCM rate than to lamotrigine in dose of 300 mg or higher.

The Efficacy of Valproic Acid in Pregnancy vs. Other Drugs

There is no high-level evidence for comparing the effectiveness of valproic acid versus alternative treatment options for JME, but valproic acid is significantly better than lamotrigine at controlling seizures in idiopathic (genetic) epilepsies in general [14]. In particular, there is substantial evidence that treatment with lamotrigine during pregnancy is associated with higher risk of seizure deterioration compared to other antiepileptic drugs including valproic acid [15] which probably is due to the pronounced gestational-related pharmacokinetic lability of lamotrigine. Use of lamotrigine during pregnancy requires therefore a close and systematic monitoring and drug adjustment throughout pregnancy for maintaining a stable plasma level which is not necessary at the same level for treatment with valproic acid. For levetiracetam, there is insufficient data about the effectiveness during pregnancy, but this drug has relative simple pharmacokinetic properties and is not expected to be associated with at higher risk of seizure deterioration than for valproic acid.

Counseling the Specific Case

Valproic acid should always be avoided during pregnancy when possible [16]. The present case has never been treated with other antiepileptic drugs and the effectiveness of levetiracetam or lamotrigine have therefore never been tested. It should be considered to switch the treatment to an alternative medication or it should be considered to decrease the dose of valproic acid to a dose under 700 mg per day. A low dose of valproic acid used in monotherapy poses a risk of MCMs that may not be significantly higher than the other drugs but it is worth to note that the differences of potential risks on neurodevelopment is relatively unknown.

It has also to be discussed that being seizure-free on a low dose of valproic acid used in monotherapy the minor differences in the teratogenic risk compared to the other antiepileptic drugs should be weighed up against the risk of seizure recurrence in case of switching the treatment. Loss of seizure control and even a single breakthrough seizure may pose serious consequences for her everyday social life. She has a full-time job and the risk of losing her ability to drive car in case of seizure recurrence may be a major issue and minimizing this risk by not changing the medication may likely be her first priority. Uncontrolled seizures can also be harmful for both the patient and the child. Studies have demonstrated that women with epilepsy have a tenfold higher risk of mortality during pregnancy compared to the women without epilepsy which stress the importance of complete seizure control [17].

Counseling the patient, it is also important to inform her that staying on valproic acid will not ensure seizure freedom during pregnancy. The elimination of valproic acid may be albeit in a minor degree affected by the pregnancy compared to the alternative drugs but therapeutic failures in pregnancy may also be caused by excessive nausea, hyperemesis, and sleep deprivation. She needs information of any aspects of her lifestyle that may affect seizure activity and those which are in her control should be addressed.

Reviewer's Comments

This case delineates a very important issue in the care of a young woman with epilepsy who is stable and seizure free and is considering pregnancy. The nature of her epilepsy syndrome, JME, is consistent with a need for lifelong therapy. The general principle in epilepsy of trying not "to rock the boat" may not apply in her circumstances where there are concerns regarding the harmful effects of the medication on her future baby. Both authors emphasize the high potential for teratogenicity of the patient's current dose of valproic acid. They both indicate that if she is to remain on the medication, then the dose should likely be reduced to under 700 mg daily to lower the potential for teratogenicity [11]. However, there is no guarantee that the patient's seizures will remain stable and controlled on this dose. Author #2 emphasizes that seizure recurrence may severely affect the patient's job, driving ability and social life and put her infant at risk if seizure breakthrough occurs during pregnancy. Author #1 suggests attempting switching the patient to an alternative therapy such as lamotrigine or levetiracetam prior to her pregnancy but the patient should be warned regarding the potential risk for losing seizure control and its consequences in her life. Both authors advise the patient to avoid sleep deprivation, alcohol consumption, and psychosocial stressors. Counselling the patient with regards to risk and benefit ratio of the above options is the key in her further management since at the end of the day, it is this patient's priorities which will shape the approach of her treating physician.

Suggested Management

1. In case of a young woman who is considering pregnancy and is seizure free on valproic acid, the high risk for potentially teratogenic side effects (10.7 %) [2] and the drug's potential for neurocognitive side effects on her future baby should be discussed.
2. If possible at all, the dose of valproic acid should be reduced to under 700 mg a day prior to pregnancy [11].
3. Consider switching to other seizure medications such as lamotrigine or levetiracetam but counsel the patient regarding the risk for losing seizure control so she can weigh the risk against the potential lower teratogenic risk to her fetus.

4. Counsel the patient regarding other controllable risk factors for seizure recurrence during pregnancy, such as inadequate sleep, alcohol consumption, and psychosocial stressors.

References

1. Calleja S, Salas-Puig J, Ribacoba R, Lahoz CH. Evolution of juvenile myoclonic epilepsy treated from the outset with sodium valproate. Seizure. 2001;10:424–7.
2. Hernandez-Diaz S, Smith CR, Shen A, Mittendorf R, Hauser WA, Yerby M, et al. Comparative safety of antiepileptic drugs during pregnancy. Neurology. 2012;78:1692–9.
3. Harden CL, Meador KJ, Pennell PB, Hauser WA, Gronseth GS, French JA, et al. Practice parameter update: management issues for women with epilepsy—focus on pregnancy (an evidence-based review): teratogenesis and perinatal outcomes: report of the Quality Standards Subcommittee and Therapeutics and Technology Assessment Subcommittee of the American Academy of Neurology and American Epilepsy Society. Neurology. 2009;73:133–41.
4. Specchio LM, Gambardella A, Giallonardo AT, Michelucci R, Specchio N, Boero G, et al. Open label, long-term, pragmatic study on levetiracetam in the treatment of juvenile myoclonic epilepsy. Epilepsy Res. 2006;71:32–9.
5. Auvin S. Treatment of myoclonic seizures in patients with juvenile myoclonic epilepsy. Neuropsychiatr Dis Treat. 2007;3:729–34.
6. Biraben A, Allain H, Scarabin JM, Schuck S, Edan G. Exacerbation of juvenile myoclonic epilepsy with lamotrigine. Neurology. 2000;55:1758.
7. McElhatton PR. The effects of benzodiazepine use during pregnancy and lactation. Reprod Toxicol. 1994;8:461–75.
8. Bilton V, Bourgeois BF. Topiramate in patients with juvenile myoclonic epilepsy. Arch Neurol. 2005;62:1705–8.
9. Margulis AV, Mitchell AA, Gilboa SM, Werler MM, Mittleman MA, Glynn RJ, et al. Use of topiramate in pregnancy and risk of oral clefts. Am J Obstet Gynecol. 2012;207:405.e1–7.
10. Kothare SV, Valencia I, Khurana DS, Hardison H, Melvin JJ, Legido A. Efficacy and tolerability of zonisamide in juvenile myoclonic epilepsy. Epileptic Disord. 2004;6:267–70.
11. Tomson T, Battino D, Bonizzoni E, Craig J, Lindhout D, Perucca E, et al. Dose-dependent teratogenicity of valproate in mono- and polytherapy: an observational study. Neurology. 2015;85:866–72.
12. Meador KJ, Baker GA, Browning N, Cohen MJ, Bromley RL, Clayton-Smith J, et al. Fetal antiepileptic drug exposure and cognitive outcomes at age 6 years (NEAD study): a prospective observational study. Lancet Neurol. 2013;12:244–52.
13. Tomson T, Battino D, Bonizzoni E, Craig J, Lindhout D, Sabers A, et al. Dose-dependent risk of malformations with antiepileptic drugs: an analysis of data from the EURAP epilepsy and pregnancy registry. Lancet Neurol. 2011;10:609–17.
14. Marson AG, Al-Kharusi AM, Alwaidh M, Appleton R, Baker GA, Chadwick DW, et al. The SANAD study of effectiveness of valproate, lamotrigine, or topiramate for generalized and unclassifiable epilepsy: an unblended randomized controlled trial. Lancet. 2007;369:1016–26.
15. Battino D, Tomson T, Bonizzoni E, Craig J, Lindhout D, Sabers A, et al. Seizure control and treatment changes in pregnancy: observations from the EURAP epilepsy pregnancy registry. Epilepsia. 2013;54:1621–7.
16. Tomson T, et al. Valproate in the treatment of epilepsy in girls and women of childbearing potential. Epilepsia. 2015;56(7):1006–1019.
17. Edey S, Moran N, Nashef L. SUDEP and epilepsy-related mortality in pregnancy. Epilepsia. 2014;55:e72–4.

Chapter 10
Epilepsy Inheritance

Madeline Fields and Mona Sazgar

Case Scenario

A 29-year-old woman has a history of epileptic seizures since age 12. Her seizures are partial onset, likely from frontal lobe origin with and without secondary generalized tonic-clonic seizures. She denies history of head injury, febrile convulsions, meningitis, or other risk factors for epilepsy. A cousin has history of convulsive seizures starting at age 16 and grew out of them by age 25 after a handful of convulsive seizures. She is worried about the risk of passing on the gene for epilepsy to her offspring and asks you whether she should refrain from having children. How do you counsel the patient?

M. Fields, M.D.
Department of Neurology, The Mount Sinai Hospital,
1 Gustave L. Levy Place, P.O. Box 1052, New York, NY 10029, USA
e-mail: madeline.fields@mssm.edu

M. Sazgar, M.D.
University of California, Irvine Medical Center,
101 The City Drive South, Pavilion I, bldg. 30, suite 123, Orange, CA 92868, USA
e-mail: msazgar@uci.edu

Commentator: C.L. Harden, M.D. (✉)
Mount Sinai Health System, Mount Sinai Beth Israel Phillips Ambulatory Care Center,
10 Union Square East, Suite 5D, New York, NY 10003, USA
e-mail: charden@chpnet.org

© Springer International Publishing Switzerland 2016
M. Sazgar, C.L. Harden (eds.), *Controversies in Caring for Women with Epilepsy*, DOI 10.1007/978-3-319-29170-3_10

Author #1's Response

Genetics is believed to play a role in most forms of epilepsy. Recent Classification by International League against Epilepsy (ILAE) changed the previous "idiopathic" category to "genetic" emphasizing the importance of genetic testing for patients and families affected by epileptic syndromes. Genetic counseling, however, is a delicate and complex matter. In counseling the patient regarding benefits of genetic testing, the potential harmful consequences such as emotional distress, potential future health and life insurance discriminations, and employment disadvantages should be addressed.

The role of inheritance in epilepsy is complex. For most people with epilepsy, the amount of increased risk is modest. The risk of epilepsy in first-degree relatives of people with epilepsy is about 2–4 times higher than the risk in general population, depending on the type of epilepsy. Studies suggest that, except in some unusual cases, the chance is less than 1 in 10 that a child of a person with epilepsy will develop epilepsy. It has been estimated that genetic epilepsy affects 0.3–0.5 % of general population. Children of one parent with genetic epilepsy have a 4–6 % risk, while children of both parents with genetic epilepsy have a 12–20 % risk [1].

Based on the mode of inheritance, the genetic epilepsies are divided into four subgroups including genetic epilepsy with Mendelian inheritance, complex inheritance, associated with cytogenetic abnormalities and Mendelian disorders in which epilepsy is one of the manifestations. A proper pedigree analysis is important in establishing the mode of inheritance in genetic epilepsies whether it is autosomal dominant, recessive, or X-linked. The complex inheritance may involve up to 50 % of genetic epilepsies [2, 3].

Autosomal dominant nocturnal frontal lobe epilepsy (ADNFLE) is the first human partial epilepsy syndrome to show autosomal dominant inheritance. In this type of epilepsy, the patient usually experiences clusters of brief nocturnal seizures, each lasting 30–40 s in duration, and with hyper motor behavior. The seizures usually occur out of light sleep and the patient remains aware during them. This seizure type is usually misdiagnosed as sleep parasomnias such as night terrors, or mistaken for behavioral and psychiatric disorders. The patient usually has normal intellect and neurologic exam as well as normal neuroimaging. The identified genes for this condition include: CHRNA4 α4 subunit (nACh receptor) [4], CHRNB2 β2 subunit (nACh receptor) [5], CHRNA2 α2 subunit (nACh receptor) [6], and DEPDC5 (a gene involved in G-protein signaling pathway loss of function) [7].

This patient's epilepsy if in fact genetic in nature is likely a form of ADNFLE. Each offspring of an affected mother has 50 % risk for inheriting the gene and with the high penetrance for this gene the chances for her children to manifest the disorder are high. Since she has already brought up the concern regarding genetic component to her epilepsy, a detailed genetic consult is warranted. Although a negative test result may provide relief to the patient and her family, there is a lot more to be discussed with the patient before offering a genetic test. It is important to point out that due to significant genetic heterogeneity, a negative test does not necessarily rule out the presence of a genetic syndrome. At our center, the patient will be referred to a geneticist who works closely with the epileptologist, for pre-test counseling and informed consent. This is important so that the patient fully understands the ramifications for her genetic testing and potential disadvantages. The shortcomings of genetic tests are explained to the patient and her family. The patient should be advised carefully regarding the potential harmful consequences of genetic testing including emotional and psychologic distress, as well as health and life insurance discrimination. She should make her own decision whether she wants to be tested. The risk of adverse effect on future insurance and employment may still be real despite the United States Genetic Information Nondiscrimination Act (GINA) in 2008, prohibiting discriminatory use of genetic information by health insurers and employers.

Once the genetic testing is performed, the post-test counseling is offered by both the geneticist and epileptologist. The epileptologist can help the patient understand what the results mean and guide this patient in her important decision whether to start a family.

Author #2's Response

An inherited component to epilepsy has been known since ancient writers first described the disease. The famous author Fyodor Dostoyevsky (*Crime and Punishment*, *The Brothers Karamazov*) was born to a father who suffered from epilepsy and whose son also had epilepsy. One of the greatest epileptologists of our time William Lennox introduced scientific methodology in the 1930s to study the inheritance of seizure disorders via twin studies. Despite tremendous developments over the last several years, progress may seem slow. This is due to the complexity of epilepsy. For one, phenotype–genotype correlations are not straightforward. The same gene mutation (i.e., sodium channel) can be associated with a benign self-limiting epilepsy syndrome (i.e., generalized epilepsy with febrile seizures plus—GEFS+) as well as one that results in severe epilepsy with intellectual impairment (i.e., severe myoclonic epilepsy of infancy—SMEI). Additionally, mutations in different genes cause syndromes that are clinically indistinguishable (i.e., febrile seizures). More likely than not the environment and genetics interact in ways we don't clearly understand. Generally speaking, the risk of inheriting epilepsy is rare. Epidemiological studies show that about 5 % of patients with epilepsy have a first-degree relative with epilepsy [8]. However, this percentage increases significantly when discussing monogenetic epilepsies (those caused by a single genetic defect), as may be the case in the patient described above.

A 'familial epilepsy syndrome' refers to people with epilepsy who have an identifiable inheritance but without neurodegenerative aspects. An example of such epilepsy is ADNFLE. This young woman's seizures are classified as partial in onset and likely originating from the frontal lobe. A subset of patients with frontal lobe seizures have ADNFLE. Scheffer et al. originally described this familial form of epilepsy in 1994 [9]. ADNFLE is the first idiopathic epilepsy to demonstrate an underlying genetic cause [4]. Idiopathic epilepsy (now called genetic) refers to patients who have epilepsy but with normal neurological examinations, normal intellect, no brain lesions, no known external cause (i.e., head trauma, meningitis) and in whom genetic factors are implicated, as in this case where other family members suffer from epilepsy as well [10].

Additional history is necessary to determine whether this woman has ADNFLE or another inheritable cause of epilepsy. The diagnosis of ADNFLE should be considered in patients with the following history: seizures with a frontal semiology, seizures predominantly during sleep, a normal neurologic examination, normal intelligence (usually), normal neuroimaging, normal interictal EEG, often normal ictal EEG (or obscured by movement and muscle artifact) and the presence of the disorder in other family members. Asking this patient if other family members suffer from nocturnal events like sleep walking (somnambulism) or night terrors can often lead to the correct diagnosis in the patient and a misdiagnosis in the family member. Note that ADNFLE may be clinically indistinguishable from those with nocturnal frontal lobe epilepsy that is not inherited [4, 9].

Genetic mutations affecting the nicotinic acetylcholine receptor (nAChR) subunits have been associated with ADNFLE. A number of different mutations have been identified. The first nAChR described was CHRNA4 [9]. Since then other nAChR subunits have been implicated including CHRNB2 and CHRNA2. Other mutations leading to a similar but sometimes more severe phenotype include a potassium channel subunit (KCNT1), a gene involved in G-protein signaling pathways (DEPDC5) and a corticotrophin-releasing hormone (CRH) gene [7, 11–14]. It should be noted that reported mutations have been identified in only a minority of patients with ADNFLE (10–15 %) [15]. This fact suggests that additional, as of yet unidentified, causative genes exist.

Due to the fact that ADNFLE is inherited in an autosomal dominant manner, most individuals with ADNFLE have an affected parent. Each offspring of a person with ADNFLE has a 50 % chance of inheriting the abnormal gene. Penetrance is estimated at 70 % (depending upon the mutation). Therefore, the chance that the offspring will manifest ADNFLE is 35 % (50 % × 70 %).

If the patient is concerned about a genetic component, it is perfectly reasonable to refer the patient to medical genetics. Specific genetic as well as genomic testing is available in general for people with epilepsy and specifically for people with ADNFLE. The best time to determine if a genetic risk is present is before the patient becomes pregnant. Identification of a specific genetic cause can help with early diagnosis, avoid future diagnostic testing, and help to select the appropriate treatment in the offspring. In this case it is the patient's choice to have genetic testing. Obtaining a genetic test and/or the results or that test may or may not determine whether the patient decides to have children but again this is the patients' decision to make. Reassuring, educating, guiding, and supporting the patient in her decision either to have genetic testing or to start a family right away is our job as physicians.

Reviewer's Comments

These two authors discussed how they would approach counseling an epilepsy patient regarding the genetics and inheritance of epilepsy. How does one undertake a discussion for which there are so few clear answers, and when the answer is clear, the consequences are so unwelcome? This seems to be the nature of genetic disorders; knowledge of their presence in a family opens a Pandora's Box of risk management, including the illegal discrimination by insurance companies, as stated by Author #1. Both authors showed amazing skill in going from the general to the particular that is from the general risk of epilepsy when there is no evidence of inheritance, to the risk for this patient, whom both authors thought had the possibility of carrying the diagnosis of Autosomal Dominant Frontal Lobe Epilepsy. Both authors showed appropriate sensitivity to the implications that genetic exploration would have for the patient and her family, and both sought partnership with medical genetics in guiding the care and counseling of this patient.

Suggested Management

1. Counseling patients on specific risks of inheritance of epilepsy should be undertaken in general terms.
2. If a genetic epilepsy syndrome is under consideration, an avenue for genetic counseling should be available at the time of testing.
3. Pre-test genetic counseling should include the potential emotional and psychological distress, life and health discrimination and other consequences.
4. Post-test counseling should be delivered by a geneticist or epileptologist to explain the results to the patient and her family.

References

1. Tafakhori A, Aghamollai V, Faghihi-Kashani S, Sarraf P, Habibi L. Epileptic syndromes: from clinic to genetic. Iran J Neurol. 2015;14:1–7.
2. Ottman R, Hirose S, Jain S, Lerche H, Lopes-Cendes I, Noebels JL, et al. Genetic testing in the epilepsies—report of the ILAE Genetics Commission. Epilepsia. 2010;51:655–70.
3. Johnson MR, Sander JW. The clinical impact of epilepsy genetics. J Neurol Neurosurg Psychiatry. 2001;70:428–30.
4. Steinlein OK, Mulley JC, Propping P, Wallace RH, Phillips HA, Sutherland GR, et al. A missense mutation in the neuronal nicotinic acetylcholine receptor alpha 4 subunit is associated with autosomal dominant nocturnal frontal lobe epilepsy. Nat Genet. 1995;11:201–3.
5. De Fusco M, Becchetti A, Patrignani A, Annesi G, Gambardella A, Quattrone A, et al. The nicotinic receptor beta 2 subunit is mutant in nocturnal frontal lobe epilepsy. Nat Genet. 2000;26:275–6.

6. Aridon P, Marini C, Di Resta C, Brilli E, De Fusco M, Politi F, et al. Increased sensitivity of the neuronal nicotinic receptor alpha 2 submit causes familial epilepsy with nocturnal wandering and ictal fear. Am J Hum Genet. 2006;79:342–50.
7. Picard F, Makrythanasis P, Navarro V, Ishida S, de Bellescize J, Ville D, et al. DEPDC5 mutations in families presenting as autosomal dominant nocturnal frontal lobe epilepsy. Neurology. 2014;82:2101–6.
8. Bianchi A, Viaggi S, Chiossi E. Family study of epilepsy in first degree relatives: data from the Italian Episcreen Study. Seizure. 2003;12:203–10.
9. Scheffer IE, Bhatia KP, Lopes-Cendes I, Fish DR, Marsden CD, Andermann F, Andermann E, Desbiens R, Cendes F, Manson JI, Berkovic S. Autosomal dominant frontal lobe epilepsy misdiagnosed as sleep disorder. Lancet. 1994;343:515–7.
10. Scheffer IE, Bhatia KP, Lopes-Cendes I, Fish DR, Marsden CD, Andermann E, Andermann F, Desbiens R, Keene D, Cendes F, Manson J, Constantinou JEC, McIntosh A, Berkovic S. Autosomal dominant nocturnal frontal lobe epilepsy: a distinctive clinical disorder. Brain. 1995;118:61–73.
11. Nobili L, Proserpio P, Combi R, Provini F, Plazzi G, Bisulli F, Tassi L, Tinuper P. Nocturnal frontal lobe epilepsy. Curr Neurol Neurosci Rep. 2014;14:424.
12. Ihida S, Picard F, Rudolf G, Noe E, Achaz G, Thomas P, Genton P, Mundwiller E, Wolff M, Marescaux C, Miles R, Baulac M, Hirsch E, Leguern E, Baulac S. Mutations of DEPDC5 cause autosomal dominant focal epilepsies. Nat Genet. 2013;45:552–5.
13. Combi R, Ferini-Strambi L, Tenchini ML. CHRNA2 mutations are rare in the NFLE population: evaluation of a large cohort of Italian patients. Sleep Med. 2009;10:139–42.
14. Sansoni V, Forcella M, Mozzi A, Fusi P, Ambrosini R, Ferini-Strambi L, Combi R. Functional characterization of a CRH missense mutation identified in an ADNFLE family. PLoS One. 2013;8:e61306.
15. Marini C, Guerrini R. The role of the nicotinic acetylcholine receptors in sleep-related epilepsy. Biochem Pharmacol. 2007;74:1308–14.

Chapter 11
Infertility and Menstrual Disorders: Seizure Medications vs. Seizures

Esther Bui and Cynthia L. Harden

Case Scenario

A 30-year-old woman has a long standing history of generalized tonic-clonic seizures since age 15. During an inpatient epilepsy monitoring, her seizures were
found to originate from dominant hemisphere frontal lobe. She has declined epilepsy surgery due to potential risks for complications. In the past she was treated
with multiple seizure medications including phenytoin, carbamazepine, topiramate,
valproic acid, and lamotrigine. Currently, she is treated on a combination of lacosamide and levetiracetam and experiences at least one break through seizure per
month. She is married and has been trying to become pregnant in the past 4 years
with no success. During her office visit, she mentions that her menstrual periods are
irregular and her gynecologist has determined that she has anovulatory cycles and
decreased chance for becoming pregnant. She also has noticed weight gain and thin-
ning of her hair, acne and excess facial hair. She is wondering whether her condition
is a result of her seizure disorder or her medications and if there is anything she can
do to improve her condition.

E. Bui, M.D., F.R.C.P.C.
Assistant Professor, Neurology Comprehensive Epilepsy Program, Toronto Western
Hospital, University of Toronto, Toronto, ON, Canada
e-mail: Esther.Bui@uhn.ca

C.L. Harden, M.D.
Mount Sinai Health System, Mount Sinai Beth Israel Phillips Ambulatory Care Center,
10 Union Square East, Suite 5D, New York, NY 10003, USA
e-mail: charden@chpnet.org

Commentator: M. Sazgar, M.D. (✉)
University of California, Irvine Medical Center,
101 The City Drive South, Pavilion I, Bldg. 30, Suite 123, Orange, CA 92868, USA
e-mail: msazgar@uci.edu

© Springer International Publishing Switzerland 2016   87
M. Sazgar, C.L. Harden (eds.), *Controversies in Caring for Women
with Epilepsy*, DOI 10.1007/978-3-319-29170-3_11

AUTHOR #1'S RESPONSE

Infertility in Women with Epilepsy

Infertility is defined as failure to conceive after >12 months of regular unprotected intercourse. Infertility in women can be caused by multiple factors such as psychosocial, hormonal, structural, and genetic factors. Both seizures and anticonvulsant medications have been implicated in infertility, with the most well-studied aspect being hormonal changes specific to women with epilepsy (WWE). It is estimated that one in three women with epilepsy have infertility compared to one in seven in the general population [1]. A recent study examining over two million people in Britain identified a 33 % reduction in fertility in WWE relative to the general population [2]. Menstrual disorders such as irregular menses and anovulatory cycles, as can be seen in polycystic ovarian syndrome (PCOS), are identified causes of infertility and are twice as common in WWE [3]. PCOS is a state of hyperandrogenic chronic anovulation diagnosed by the presence of two of the following: polycystic ovaries, hyperandrogenism, and ovulatory dysfunction. It affects 10–20 % of WWE compared to 5–6 % of the general population [4].

Normal Hypothalamic–Pituitary–Ovarian Axis

Estrogen and progesterone are the two major sex hormones produced by ovaries. Upstream, gonadotropin-releasing hormone (GnRH) is secreted by the hypothalamus resulting in release of follicular stimulating hormone (FSH) by the pituitary. FSH stimulates follicular development in the ovaries with follicles secreting estrogen. Rising estrogen levels stimulate a surge in pituitary luteinizing hormone (LH) through feedback mechanisms (Fig. 11.1) resulting in ovulation. After ovulation, the remaining corpus luteum secretes progesterone. If pregnancy does not occur, the corpus luteum regresses and estrogen and progesterone levels fall. Women with normal fertility have hormone levels within an established range throughout their menstrual cycle. In contrast, Thomas et al. identified a distinct hormonal profile in WWE consisting of higher levels of LH and dehydroepiandrostenedione (DHEA), the latter an important precursor to testosterone in addition to lower levels of progesterone supporting a hormonal basis for increased infertility in WWE [5].

Seizures and Infertility

Psychosocial Impact

WWE face challenges associated with the impact of seizure itself including stigma, lower socioeconomic status, comorbid depression, and anxiety, in addition to lower marriage or cohabitation rates, all potentially contributing to lower fertility rates

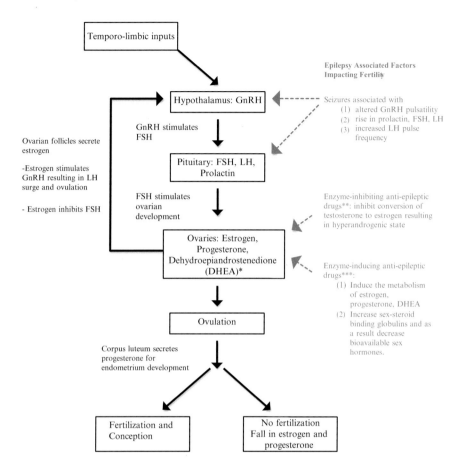

*DHEA also produced in adrenal glands
**Valproic acid
***Phenytoin, Carbamazepine, Phenobarbital

Fig. 11.1 Hypothalamic–pituitary–ovarian axis

[6]. However, even among married people with epilepsy, fertility rates remain lower than the general population. In addition to decreased libido and sexual dysfunction observed in WWE, neuroendocrine factors likely also contribute [7–9].

Neuroendocrine Impact

Seizures may disrupt the balance of sex hormones through temporolimbic connections to the hypothalamus and pituitary. It is recognized that prolactin, FSH, and LH levels rise significantly following generalized and complex partial seizures [10]. In addition to elevated hormone levels, an altered *pattern* of secretion has been observed. Bilo identified an increased LH pulse frequency in untreated WWE [11]. Of interest not only ictal but also interictal discharges have been associated with an increase in GnRH pulsatility [12].

Additional studies have delineated distinct forms of infertility based on seizure type. Right temporal lobe seizures have been associated with hypothalamic amenorrhea (dysfunction of hypothalamic GnRH secretion) whereas left temporal seizures have been associated with PCOS though interestingly this lateralization was not observed in non-temporal foci [13]. To support the impact of seizures on fertility, following successful temporal lobe surgery birth rates have been observed to increase suggesting a therapeutic role of seizure reduction in fertility [14].

Antiepileptic Drugs and Infertility

Antiepileptic drugs (AEDs) particularly polytherapy is associated with higher rates of infertility. WWE not on AEDs had an observed infertility rate of 7.1 % whereas WWE on 1 AED, 2 AEDs, and 3 or more AEDs had observed infertility rates of 31.8 %, 40.7 %, and 60.3 %, respectively [15]. Key differences in how AEDs impact fertility have been identified, distinguishing enzyme-inhibiting from enzyme-inducing AEDs.

Enzyme-Inhibiting Antiepileptic Drugs

Though PCOS has been reported in association to seizures, independent of AEDs [11] it has also been associated with anticonvulsant medication, specifically valproate. Valproate inhibits cytochrome P450 enzymes and as such inhibits the conversion of testosterone to estrogen resulting in a hyperandrogenic state. In a European study involving 72 WWE and 52 control subjects, 70 % of WWE treated with valproate had polycystic ovaries and/or hyperandrogenism compared to 19 % of controls [16]. Controversy from this study lies in the reporting of polycystic ovaries, which in isolation does not constitute a diagnosis of PCOS and may not be clinically significant. In addition, it remains to be clarified whether valproate directly via enzyme inhibition or indirectly via weight gain and insulin resistance results in the observed hyperandrogenic state.

Enzyme-Inducing Antiepileptic Drugs

In contrast, enzyme-inducing AEDs such as Carbamazepine have been associated with a lower rate of PCOS [17]. However, they may contribute to infertility by other methods including observed lower levels of estrogen, progesterone, DHEA and increases in sex steroid-binding globulin levels, the latter decreasing the bio-availability of sex hormones and plausibly impacting fertility [18].

Newer Anticonvulsants

Less is known about the newer agents, though observations have been made on lamotrigine. Lamotrigine when compared to valproate had significantly lower rates of ovulatory dysfunction (54 % versus 38 %) and PCOS (9 % versus 2 %) [19]. In one animal model study using rats, an 8-week course of topiramate and gabapentin therapy was associated with altered hormonal levels and menses postulated to be through the GnRH pulse generator in the hypothalamus [20].

Premature Menopause

A less studied reproductive aspect in WWE is early menopause. As many women choose to start families later in life, this may be an increasingly important factor to consider. Most women experience menopause between 48 and 55 years of age. The median age of menopause in WWE is 47 versus 51.4 in the general population [21]. Early menopause is identified at a higher rate in WWE than controls 14 % versus 4 %, respectively [22]. Though not observed in Klein's study, a separate study identified greater lifetime seizures and polytherapy to be correlated with earlier menopause [23].

Review of Case

In our patient, once male factor infertility has been ruled out, by definition she has infertility. She has multiple risk factors for infertility including intractable seizures and polytherapy. Both play important and likely interrelated roles in affecting fertility. Notably she presents with clinical features suggestive of a hyperandrogenic state such as PCOS. From the literature, factors associated with PCOS include left temporal lobe seizures and valproate. However, the weight gain associated with anticonvulsant likely also contributes.

I would tell her that no current fertility-related data is available for newer AEDs such as lacosamide and levetiracetam. To confirm my clinical suspicion of PCOS, you discuss with her family doctor regarding hormone levels including day 3 LH, FSH, and testosterone levels in addition to considering a pelvic ultrasound for polycystic ovaries. I recommend a referral to a reproductive specialist for a formal opinion. In the interim, I would titrate her anticonvulsant medication to optimize seizure control and re-discuss the role of epilepsy surgery particularly if her quality of life is significantly impacted by her current seizure frequency. If the patient is content with my comprehensive explanation and plan, I will see her for follow-up after the above investigations.

Recommendations

- Take a reproductive history in all WWE of child-bearing age
- Identify risk factors for infertility in WWE [4]:
    - Poorly controlled epilepsy
    - Polytherapy
    - Valproic acid
- Clinically assess for endocrine dysfunction (See Fig. 11.2):
    - Irregular menses, male pattern baldness, obesity, hirsutism, galactorrhea
- Consider additional tests [24]:
    - Day 3 of menstrual cycle: LH, FSH, Testosterone: if elevated LH/FSH ratio >2 or elevated Testosterone >2.5 nmol/L suggests PCOS
    - Midluteal progesterone: if low levels suggest anovulation*

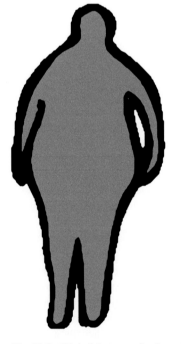

- Male-pattern baldness

- Acne

- Obstructive sleep apnea

- Excessive hair growth (face, chest, back, buttock)

- Weight gain

- Polycystic ovaries

- Irregular or absent menses

- Glucose intolerance

- Dyslipidemia

Fig. 11.2 Clinical features of polycystic ovarian syndrome

- Dehydroepiandrostenedione (DHEA) levels
- Prolactin, Glucose, Insulin levels
- Pelvic ultrasound
- Pituitary imaging

• Consider referral to reproductive specialist

   *luteal phase being days 15–28 in a 28-day menstrual cycle

AUTHOR # 2'S RESPONSE

This is an interesting and difficult case wherein a young woman is struggling with several difficult medical problems. They are (1) the disease of epilepsy, (2) the disease of infertility and (3) quite likely the syndrome of polycystic ovaries (PCOS) and its associated endocrine dysfunction. The question to the practitioner is whether her "condition" is a result of her seizure disorder or her antiseizure medications and if there is anything she can do to improve her "condition."

First of all, I would ask her exactly what she means by her "condition," specifically if she means her inability to conceive, her recent hyperandrogenism, or her seizure disorder. She probably means the former two issues, whereas, as an epilepsy neurologist, I am most capable of helping to improve her epilepsy rather than the other two problems, and of note, her seizures are not at all well-controlled. She has already "declined" surgery although she is certainly in a medication-resistant category of epilepsy. I would take her decision personally as a failure on my part to educate her regarding the risk versus benefit balance between at least exploring the chance of successful epilepsy surgery compared to continued medical treatment. It is quite likely however, that the desire for children is the overriding concern for this patient and this is what she wants to discuss.

There are certainly associations between having epilepsy and bearing fewer children [25] and between epilepsy and PCOS [26]. In a study published from the Finnish Birth Cohort [25], persons with "active epilepsy" did not produce live births at the expected comparator rate, whereas those with well-controlled epilepsy bore children at the same rates as the general population. The authors stated that epilepsy patients with disability and severe comorbid conditions did not produce children and for the most part accounted for the baby gap between epilepsy patients and the general population. In other words, if the epilepsy is well-controlled and the patient is presumably functioning independently in society, there is a good chance that offspring will follow at an expected rate.

There are also associations between infertility and taking several of the strong enzyme-inducing antiseizure medications [15]. Dr. Sanjeev Thomas within his database from the Kerala province reported that WWE taking phenobarbital and phenytoin particularly as polytherapy produced significantly less children. They also noted decreased education as an independent risk factor for infertility and exactly how this piece fits into the puzzle I am unsure. For our discussion, our patient is not taking these medications and presumably the exposure was in the remote past.

Valproate use has been clearly associated with PCOS [27]. But again, her exposure was in the past and the adverse effects of valproate (and carbamazepine) on reproductive hormone profiles are reversible when the drug is stopped, as shown by Lossius et al. in 2007 [28]. There have been hints that PCOS is overrepresented in the epilepsy population even outside of valproate use; however, this evidence is slim, especially given that PCOS in its multiple variations is also very common, likely present in 15–20 % of women of reproductive potential. Therefore, the association between epilepsy and PCOS is not robust enough to be considered causal, that is, epilepsy has not been shown to cause PCOS, and the vast majority of women with PCOS do not have epilepsy.

Finally, infertility is not the same as not bearing children. Many persons with epilepsy, due to their comorbidities and disabilities, will not bear children; a proportion more will choose not to because of the perceived risks involved, including that their own children will suffer from epilepsy. This is where further education regarding the actual risks surrounding pregnancy and childbearing may be helpful toward making sure patients are making decisions informed by facts and not fear, since the risks are mostly low.

The World Health Organization defines infertility as "a disease of the reproductive system defined by the failure to achieve a clinical pregnancy after 12 months or more of regular unprotected sexual intercourse." The patient has a risk of infertility based solely upon being age 30 of at least 10 % [29]. I cannot counsel this 30-year-old patient in good faith that any of her reproductive problems are caused by or even significantly contributed to by epilepsy or epilepsy treatments. All three medical problems are common, and yes, there are threads that may join them, but they could also occur independently. There is really no counseling advantage to telling an already distraught young woman that her seizure disorder is causing her to become infertile and hirsute. She should be reassured that the medications for seizures currently in use and those used in the past are not contributing to the reproductive problems. The last thing I would want this patient with severe refractory epilepsy who has frequent generalized tonic-clonic seizures to do is to taper or stop her medications because she thinks that doing so may improve fertility.

Basically, she likely has two treatable illnesses, and as an epilepsy neurologist, I am responsible for one of them. First, she should be counseled on further medical treatments for epilepsy and the surgical issue, including options such as the vagus nerve stimulator, should be gently re-addressed. She should be counseled that when she gets pregnant, and I would emphasize "when," because she is only 30 years old and there is a lot of time to work with the fertility problem; it would be greatly, vastly preferable to have the seizures under control. Second, she probably has infertility from the very common syndrome of PCOS. This is also manageable and pregnancy is quite possible under the care of a reproductive endocrinologist.

Overall, this patient, who has lived for a long time with probably at least some degree of fear, shame, worry, blame, and dread about having seizures and the consequences of seizures and of taking the medications, should be reassured. She should be reassured that the epilepsy did not cause her reproductive problems and that PCOS along with trouble conceiving unfortunately happens to many, many women who do not have epilepsy. She should be reassured that her health care providers have expertise to help her, and share with her the fervent hope of getting better and the heartbreaking anxiety of setbacks along the way.

Reviewer's Comments

This is a very delicate and difficult case scenario, with an emotionally tasking problem regarding a woman with epilepsy who is unsuccessfully trying to become pregnant for 4 years. The two authors are handling the counseling from two separate angles. Both authors are aware of the data that may link the patient's lack of ability to conceive, anovulatory cycles and endocrine problems to her uncontrolled epilepsy and/or seizure medications. Author #2 argues that not bearing children does not equal infertility and can be due to many reasons. She gives the patient the benefit of the doubt that her infertility might be unrelated to her epilepsy and seizure medications. In other words she raises the possibility that many infertility problems can be addressed and cured by an expert reproductive endocrinologist. She sees no benefit in letting the patient worry about possibility of her seizures or seizure medications contributing to the problem. The first author emphasizes the data regarding seizures and seizure medications associated with infertility and that menstrual disorders such as irregular menses and anovulatory cycles are twice as common in WWE. She explains that epileptiform discharges can alter the level of sex hormones at the hypothalamic and pituitary level, disrupting the menstrual cycle and affecting fertility. Both authors agree that with the patient's current medications, there is no sufficient data to suggest their role in patient's infertility.

Both authors agree in aggressively treating the patient's epilepsy and re-opening the dialog about epilepsy surgery and/or vagus nerve stimulator. This is partly based on population studies such as the Northern Finland Birth Cohort 1966 which found that well-controlled epilepsy patients in remission have the same number of children as the control group. "Active" epilepsy requiring medications in adulthood, on the other hand, was a risk factor for lower birth rate. In other words, the emphasis is on what an epileptologist or treating physician can do to fully control the patient's seizures and enhance her chance for fertility. The treating physician should collaborate with the reproductive specialist to address the underlying cause and treatment for the patient's unsuccessful attempts to become pregnant.

Suggested Management

In a patient with signs and symptoms of reproductive dysfunction:

1. Know the signs and symptoms such as irregular menses, male pattern baldness, obesity, hirsutism, galactorrhea

2. Know the risk factors of PCOS including uncontrolled seizures, polytherapy, and certain seizure medications including valproate, carbamazepine, phenobarbital, and phenytoin
3. Counsel the patient regarding the data that controlled epilepsy can contribute to better chance of achieving pregnancy
4. Explore all the options including medical and surgical ones to achieve seizure freedom
5. Reproductive specialists, including an endocrinologist to investigate the possibility of PCOS and other reversible endocrine dysfunctions and fertility specialist to identify causes of infertility

References

1. Herzog AG. Menstrual disorders in women with epilepsy. Neurology. 2006;66 Suppl 3:S23–8.
2. Wallace H, Shorvon S, Tallis R. Age-specific incidence and prevalence rates of treated epilepsy in an unselected population of 2,052,922 and age-specific fertility rates of women with epilepsy. Lancet. 1998;352:1970–3.
3. Herzog AG, Friedman MN. Menstrual cycle interval and ovulation in women with localization-related epilepsy. Neurology. 2001;57:2133–5.
4. Herzog AG. Disorders of reproduction in patients with epilepsy: primary neurological mechanisms. Seizure. 2008;17:101–10.
5. Thomas SV, Sarma PS, Nirmala C, et al. Women with epilepsy and infertility have different reproductive hormone profile than others. Ann Indian Acad Neurol. 2013;16(4):544–8.
6. Dansky LV, Andermann E, Andermann F. Marriage and fertility in epileptic patients. Epilepsia. 1980;21:261–71.
7. Weber MO, Hauser WA, Ottman R, Annegers JF. Fertility in persons with epilepsy: 1935-1974. Epilepsia. 1986;27(6):746–52.
8. Schupf N, Ottman R. Reproduction among individuals with idiopathic/cryptogenic epilepsy: risk factors for reduced fertility in marriage. Epilepsia. 1996;37(9):833–40.
9. Morrell MJ, Flynn KL, Doñe S, et al. Sexual dysfunction, sex steroid hormone abnormalities, and depression in women with epilepsy treated with antiepileptic drugs. Epilepsy Behav. 2005;6(3):360–5.
10. Bauer J. Epilepsy and prolactin in adults: a clinical review. Epilepsy Res. 1996;24:1–7.
11. Bilo L, Meo R, Valentino R, et al. Characterization of reproductive endocrine disorders in women with epilepsy. J Clin Endocrinol Metab. 2001;86:2950–6.
12. Mahesh VB, Brann DW. Regulation of the pre-ovulatory gonadotropin surge by endogenous steroids. Steroids. 1998;63:616–29.
13. Herzog AG. A relationship between particular reproductive endocrine disorders and the laterality of epileptiform discharges in women with epilepsy. Neurology. 1993;43:1907–10.
14. Baird AD, Wilson SJ, Bladin PF, et al. Sexual outcome after epilepsy surgery. Epilepsy Behav. 2003;4:268–78.
15. Sukumaran SC, Sarma PS, Thomas SV. Polytherapy increases the risk of infertility in women with epilepsy. Neurology. 2010;75(15):1351–5.
16. Isojarvi JL, Tauboll E, Pakarinen AJ. Altered ovarian function and cardiovascular risk factors in valproate-treated women. Am J Med. 2001;111(4):290–6.
17. Hamed SA, Hamed EA, Shokry M, et al. The reproductive conditions and lipid profile in females with epilepsy. Acta Neurol Scand. 2007;115:12–22.
18. Isojarvi JI. Serum steroid hormones and pituitary function in female epileptic patients during carbamazepine therapy. Epilepsia. 1990;31(4):438–45.

19. Morrell MJ, Hayes FJ, Sluss PM, et al. Hyperandrogenism, ovulatory dysfunction, and poly-cystic ovary syndrome with valproate versus lamotrigine. Ann Neurol. 2008;64(2):200–11.
20. Kumar S, Kaur G. Second generation anti-epileptic drugs adversely affect reproductive func-tions in young non-epileptic female rats. Eur Neuropsychopharmacol. 2014;24(10):1709–18.
21. Pennell PB. Hormonal aspects of epilepsy. Neurol Clin. 2009;27(4):941–65.
22. Klein P, Serje A, Pezzullo JC. Premature ovarian failure in women with epilepsy. Epilepsia. 2001;42:1584–9.
23. Harden CL, Koppel BS, Herzog AG, et al. Seizure frequency is associated with age of meno-pause in women with epilepsy. Neurology. 2003;61:451–5.
24. Bauer J, Isojarvi JI, Herzog AG, et al. Reproductive dysfunction in women with epilepsy: recom-mendations for evaluation and management. J Neurol Neurosurg Psychiatry. 2002;73(2):121–5.
25. Löfgren EL, Pouta A, von Wendt L, Tapanainen J, Isojärvi JI, Järvelin MR. Epilepsy in the northern Finland birth cohort 1966 with special reference to fertility. Epilepsy Behav. 2009;14(1):102–7.
26. Zhou JQ, Zhou LM, Chen LJ, Han JD, Wang Q, Fang ZY, Chen ZY, Ling S. Polycystic ovary syndrome in patients with epilepsy: a study in 102 Chinese women. Seizure. 2012;21(9):729–33.
27. Hu X, Wang J, Dong W, Fang Q, Hu L, Liu C. A meta-analysis of polycystic ovary syndrome in women taking valproate for epilepsy. Epilepsy Res. 2011;97(1–2):73–82.
28. Lossius MI, Taubøll E, Mowinckel P, Mørkrid L, Gjerstad L. Reversible effects of antiepilep-tic drugs on reproductive endocrine function in men and women with epilepsy—a prospective randomized double-blind withdrawal study. Epilepsia. 2007;48(10):1875–82.
29. Tietze C. Reproductive span and the rate of conception among Hutterite women. Fertil Steril. 1957;8:89–97.

Chapter 12
Ever Advise Against Pregnancy?

Mona Sazgar and Frank J.E. Vajda

Case Scenario

A 38-year-old woman has posttraumatic medically refractory epilepsy in the past 2 years. Her epilepsy monitoring is consistent with multifocal seizure foci. She is on a combination of oxcarbazepine, lamotrigine, topiramate, and vagal nerve stimulator and continues to experience at least one episode of convulsive seizure per week. She had got married a year before her head injury and is considering pregnancy. Would you recommend against pregnancy in this case?

AUTHOR #1'S RESPONSE

This is a very difficult case of drug-resistant posttraumatic multifocal epilepsy and exceedingly difficult to render seizure free, quite apart from the aspects of desiring to achieve a pregnancy.

M. Sazgar, M.D.
University of California, Irvine Medical Center,
101 The City Drive South, Pavilion I, Bldg. 30, Suite 123, Orange, CA 92868, USA
e-mail: msazgar@uci.edu

F.J.E. Vajda, MB, BS, MD, FRCP, FRACP
Department of Medicine and Neuroscience, Royal Melbourne Hospital,
Melbourne, VIC 3052, Australia
e-mail: vajda@netspace.net; Frank.Vajda@mh-org.au

Commentator: C.L. Harden, M.D. (✉)
Mount Sinai Health System, Mount Sinai Beth Israel Phillips Ambulatory Care Center,
10 Union Square East, Suite 5D, New York, NY 10003, USA
e-mail: charden@chpnet.org

© Springer International Publishing Switzerland 2016
M. Sazgar, C.L. Harden (eds.), *Controversies in Caring for Women with Epilepsy*, DOI 10.1007/978-3-319-29170-3_12

The patient is receiving three second-generation drugs, plus a vagal nerve stimulator and still experiences one convulsive seizure per week. Despite this I respect her wishes to have a baby, even if it means admitting her to hospital and monitoring her throughout a large part of her pregnancy. I would inform her of the risks, of the possible complications of pregnancy, of seizures, and physical teratogenicity plus cognitive and behavior challenges to the baby posed by the medications. If she is cognitively normal and can evaluate the explanations about the various risks and also has financial and social support to be able to become a parent successfully and care for her baby, I would support her wishes.

She has no other children, so she would be even more anxious to conceive than a multiparous woman. We do not wish to increase her drug load, but the regimen may be optimized.

The first question is whether she is compliant with medication and if drugs she is currently taking are given in adequate doses. This could be assessed by serum therapeutic level assays [1]. If the doses are inadequate, they could be increased to the maximum tolerated. If compliance is uncertain, this could be tested in hospital. The medications she is taking may not be the most appropriate, but we need to have access to the past history of treatment. Merely adding more drugs is unlikely to help [2]. The older antiepileptic agents may provide better control as there is some evidence that of the newer AEDs only levetiracetam is equally efficacious, compared to the traditional drugs [3]. We need to know if she had already failed levetiracetam, If not, I suggest introducing levetiracetam in a small dose carefully noting the immediate possible benefit on seizure control, which give an indication that this approach is correct. Later, increase the doses of this drug but in parallel reduce some of the others.

I would start reducing lamotrigine, which may be the least effective drug, even more so as it is particularly difficult to use in pregnancy—if that were to occur—for a number of reasons viz. increased glucuridination, and thus an increased clearance, with a consequent need to adjust doses of lamotrigine in each trimester and reduction to pre-pregnancy dose levels on delivery. I would replace lamotrigine with levetiracetam in a planned manner using lower doses of levetiracetam initially than recommended, I would also look critically at topiramate intake and note whether the doses given thus far were limited by intolerance, compliance or lack of effect and adjust as required. I would not like her to continue on a high dose of topiramate in pregnancy, as this drug also shows a dose-related teratogenicity based on relatively recent evidence [4]. Oxcarbazepine may be continued as it is less of an enzyme inducer than CBZ, and assuming hyponatraemia is not a problem here, there is no class I evidence of its synergism with levetiracetam. The manipulations thus far would take several weeks to stabilize. Meantime I would prescribe folic acid 0.4–5 mg per day in anticipation of being able to achieve pregnancy. The vagus nerve stimulator may be continued, until there is evidence of a marked improvement of seizure control and even beyond it, if necessary. Clobazam added to the regimen may be of significant benefit.

If no significant improvement were to occur I would ask her to be reviewed by a most eminent epilepsy surgery programme, to see if all seizures arise from the same area of the brain and although multifocal, whether surgery could conceivably offer a significant benefit making her seizure-free. If she were rendered seizure-free, we know that a year of seizure freedom may improve the outlook for a successful course of pregnancy, the improvement being of the order of 70 %, but at the age of 38 there may be age-related reasons for not deferring pregnancy.

Major lifestyle recommendations should be advised—viz. minimizing stress, advising adequate sleep, avoidance of dehydration, overhydration, alcohol, excessive visual stimulation, and excitement, such as sporting events. Depending on progress and seizure control, I would be supportive of her getting pregnant , pointing out the risk associated with seizures and also that medications themselves pose a risk, but risks exist more along the lines of injury, rather than teratogenicity as the drugs mentioned are not highly teratogenic, at least compared valproate or cytotoxic drugs . One additional problem which cannot be expected to be overcome is the issue of polytherapy and its effect on cognition. This may be unavoidable and may relate to drug exposure over the whole of pregnancy. This is a calculated risk for the patient, and needs full explanation [5].

- In summary, I would encourage the lady to have a baby, but try to control seizures first.
- Explain that seizure freedom offers best chance for uneventful and good pregnancy.
- Alter medications.

  - Use LEV, remove LTG and probably TPM. Slow changeover.
  - Admit to hospital to test serum levels and assess compliance.
  - May add clobazam in small gradual increments as an adjuvant drug.

- Check past drug history, to see if any of the traditional drugs were tried and found ineffective or not.
- Review the efficacy of VNS.
- Refer to an established and experienced Neurosurgical Programme, and even consider hemispherectomy if necessary.
- If all above measures fail, explain the risks, but still respect her wishes.
- We know that in pregnancy many, possibly over 30 % of patients, improve with regard to seizure control. We also know that addition of AEDs to a current regimen is unlikely to influence seizure control, but in this case the manipulation consists of employing possibly more effective drugs and reducing those which failed up to this time, thus attempting to individualize therapy.

AUTHOR #2'S RESPONSE

The majority of women with epilepsy give birth to normal, healthy children. There is a modestly increased risk of major congenital malformations, about 1.5–2-fold, among offspring of women treated for epilepsy during their pregnancy. The first cases of increased risk for congenital malformation in children of women with epilepsy were reported as early as 1960s [6]. Since then, numerous studies and recent multiple pregnancy registries have confirmed the increased teratogenic risk to the babies born to mothers with epilepsy taking anticonvulsant therapy during their pregnancies. A meta-analysis of 59 studies in the literature by Meador and colleagues systematically reviewed the risk of AEDs during pregnancy. They estimated the overall prevalence of congenital malformation in children of women with epilepsy to be increased three times compared with healthy women [7]. This risk could be due to AEDs or other factors related to maternal epilepsy. In a pooled analysis of data from 26 studies Shorvon et al. reported the overall malformation rate in children of women with epilepsy to be 6.1 % as compared with 2.8 % in untreated women with epilepsy or 2.2 % in general healthy women population [8].

A recent meta-analysis of women exposed to topiramate during their pregnancy confirms that first-trimester exposure to topiramate is associated with a sixfold increased risk of oral clefts [9]. In March 2011, the FDA moved topiramate to a category D pregnancy label. In the North American AED Pregnancy Registry (NAAPR), lamotrigine monotherapy during pregnancy was associated with a 1.9 % risk for malformation in the fetus [10]. Data on other newer AEDs are insufficient but so far do not indicate an alarmingly high risk with gabapentin, oxcarbazepine, and levetiracetam. There are only isolated case reports in the literature indicating possible safety of vagal nerve stimulator in pregnant patients [11, 12].

Polytherapy in women with epilepsy carries a higher risk of fetal congenital malformation estimated at 6.8 % as compared with monotherapy with a risk around 4 % [8]. The teratogenic effects of AEDs appear to be dose dependent. There is an increased risk due to higher doses of valproate, carbamazepine, phenobarbital, and lamotrigine. The European epilepsy and pregnancy registry (EURAP) partially addressed the question of dose-dependent risk of malformation with antiepileptic drugs [13]. A dose of 300 mg or lower lamotrigine was associated with a risk of 2 % but higher doses than 300 mg of lamotrigine monotherapy was associated with a risk of 4.5 %. They found a much more significant dose dependent increased teratogenicity risk with carbamazepine at higher than 400 mg, phenobarbital at higher than 150 mg and valproic acid at higher than 700 mg daily dose.

Our patient presented above has a difficult case of medically refractory epilepsy and unlikely to be an epilepsy surgery candidate due to multifocal epilepsy. The true multifocality of her epilepsy should be established through inpatient continuous video-EEG monitoring and with confirming that in fact the seizures are originating from independent foci. Otherwise the possibility of epilepsy surgery candidacy cannot be entirely ruled out. I assume that is already the case and the reason she was considered for VNS. My first step is to establish patient's compliance with medications and the fact that her seizure recurrence is not due to missing medications and intolerable side effects. If in fact her seizures are due to noncompliance, I will attempt to identify the medication which is not well tolerated and replace it with an AED that she tolerates better, keeping the pregnancy safety profile of the medication in mind. Levetiracetam may be a candidate medication in that case. I will do every attempt to simplify her seizure medications if at all possible. I will start with tapering her off topiramate which is a pregnancy category D medication. Lamotrigine and oxcarbazepine based on the above presented and available data have better safety profile during pregnancy. I will make sure the patient is taking folic acid and prenatal vitamins. I will also try to find the optimal VNS setting to control her seizures. My extensive prenatal counselling will include explanation that, despite all the risks described above; the majority of patients with epilepsy give birth to normal healthy babies. As long as she is making an informed decision, I will fully support her decision to become pregnant and start a family. I will involve a high-risk obstetrician in her care. I will make sure her baseline AED levels are known and will follow them closely during pregnancy and adjust the dose if necessary. Once pregnant, she will be offered prenatal screening tests to detect any possible fetal congenital malformations including serum AFPs, amniocentesis and detailed ultrasound at 16–17 weeks of pregnancy. Her care will involve close follow-up and communication between her epileptologist and high-risk obstetrician throughout her pregnancy to ensure the safety and health of both mother and baby.

Reviewer's Comments

This is certainly a case where some physicians would "just say 'no'!" They would advise against pregnancy for now and perhaps forever for this patient with treatment-resistant epilepsy due to structural brain injury secondary to head trauma. The experts herein did not advise this. They both demonstrated extreme empathy for the patient and offered all forms of available support to optimize the pregnancy outcome, such as instituting folic acid use and referring to a high-risk obstetrician. Keep in mind, both authors have their eyes open; Author #2 in particular discussed the teratogenic risks of polypharmacy and of epilepsy itself. Both authors would undertake efforts to reduce seizure frequency and both suggested levetiracetam as a medication of choice to try.

What does this imply for the complex physician–patient relationship? For this difficult patient, experienced and thoughtful epilepsy doctors understand the nuances of the risks she faces, and know that some treatment-associated risks are greater than others and further can convey that there is never a pregnancy that is without risks. They also have an appreciation for the importance and deep meaning of the conscious decision on the part of this patient to try to have a child. Therefore, instead of warning her against it and emphasizing the risks, they are willing to dig in and optimize her care by whatever means necessary, starting from assessing medication compliance, through medication changes to evaluating for epilepsy surgery. As usual in medicine, there is not just one correct course of action. But there is a course of action here that is perhaps more informed and more compassionate than another. This course of action requires more engagement of the patient into an informed partnership, more decision-making, and overall, more work and risk for the physician. These experts, Authors #1 and #2, certainly believe that it is worth it.

Suggested Management

1. In case of women with medically refractory epilepsy on polypharmacy, pregnancy is not completely ruled out.
2. Review lifestyle contributors to seizure occurrence and advise them to modify their risk factors for seizure recurrence.
3. Undertake renewed efforts to improve seizure control by medical and surgical intervention if needed.
4. Follow them closely during pregnancy and adjust their medication levels.
5. In collaboration with high-risk obstetrician offer prenatal screening tests to detect any possible fetal congenital malformations including serum AFPs, amniocentesis, and detailed ultrasound at 16–17 weeks of pregnancy
6. Start folic acid 1–4 mg per day and refer to high-risk obstetrical practice.

References

1. Tomson T, Landmark CJ, Battino D. Antiepileptic drug treatment in pregnancy: changes in drug disposition and their clinical implications. Epilepsia. 2013;54(3):405.
2. Kwan P, Sperling MR. Refractory seizures. Try additional antiepileptic drugs (after two have failed) or go directly to early surgery evaluation? Epilepsia. 2009;50 Suppl 8:57–62.
3. Vajda FJE, O'Brien TJ, Lander CM, Graham J, Eadie MJ. The efficacy of the newer antiepileptic drugs in controlling seizures in pregnancy. Epilepsia. 2014;55(8):1229–34.
4. Vajda FJE, O'Brien TJ, Graham J, Lander CM, Eadie MJ. Associations between particular types of fetal malformation and antiepileptic drug exposure in utero. Acta Neurol Scand. 2013;128:228–34.
5. Palac S, Meador KJ. Antiepileptic drugs and neurodevelopment: an update. Curr Neurol Neurosci Rep. 2011;11:423–7.
6. Meadow SR. Anticonvulsant drugs and congenital abnormalities. Lancet. 1968;2:1296.
7. Meador K, Reynolds MW, Crean S, Fahrbach K, Probst C. Pregnancy outcomes in women with epilepsy: a systematic review and meta-analysis of published pregnancy registries and cohorts. Epilepsy Res. 2008;81:1–13.
8. Shorvon SD, Tomson T, Cock HR. The management of epilepsy during pregnancy—progress is painfully slow. Epilepsia. 2009;50:973–4.
9. Alsaad AM, Chaudhry SA, Koren G. First trimester exposure to topiramate and the risk of oral clefts in the offspring: a systematic review and meta-analysis. Reprod Toxicol. 2015;53:45–50.
10. Hernandez-Diaz S, Smith CR, Shen A, Mittendorf R, Hauser WA, Yerby M, et al. Comparative safety of antiepileptic drugs during pregnancy. Neurology. 2012;78:1692–9.
11. Husain MM, Stegman D, Trevino K. Pregnancy and delivery while receiving vagus nerve stimulation for the treatment of major depression: a case report. Ann Gen Psychiatry. 2005;4:16.
12. Salerno G, Passamonti C, Cecchi A, Zamponi N. Vagus nerve stimulation during pregnancy: an instructive case. Childs Nerv Syst. 2015 Sep 9. [Epub ahead of print].
13. Tomson T, Battino D, Bonizzoni E, Craig J, Lindhout D, Sabers A, et al. Dose-dependent risk of malformations with antiepileptic drugs: an analysis of data from the EURAP epilepsy and pregnancy registry. Lancet Neurol. 2011;10:609–17.

Part III
Pregnancy/Breast Feeding

Chapter 13
New Onset Seizures During Pregnancy

Chellamani Harini and Lilit Mnatsakanyan

Case Scenario

A 24-year-old pregnant woman (G1P0) presents with new onset epilepsy. She found out about her pregnancy after her first witnessed generalized tonic-clonic seizure when she ended up in the emergency room and beta HCG was sent for by the emergency room physician. The week before her visit to your office, she experienced a second unprovoked generalized tonic-clonic seizure out of sleep which was accompanied with tongue laceration. Both seizures were witnessed by her husband who accompanies her to this consultation visit. She is at her 5th week of gestation and has no known risk factors for epilepsy. Her MRI of brain is within normal limits. Her EEG shows left temporal sharp waves potentiated during sleep. What is the treatment you suggest? How do you counsel the patient if she is hesitant or decides not to take seizure medications during her pregnancy?

C. Harini, M.D.
Division of Neurophysiology, Boston Children's Hospital,
Fegan 9, 300, Longwood Avenue, Boston, MA 02115, USA
e-mail: chellamani.harini@childrens.harvard.edu

L. Mnatsakanyan, M.D.
Department of Neurology, University of California Irvine Medical Center,
101 The City Dr South, Orange, CA 92868, USA
e-mail: mnatsakl@uci.edu

Commentator: M. Sazgar, M.D. (✉)
University of California, Irvine Medical Center,
101 The City Drive South, Pavilion I, Bldg. 30, Suite 123, Orange, CA 92868, USA
e-mail: msazgar@uci.edu

© Springer International Publishing Switzerland 2016
M. Sazgar, C.L. Harden (eds.), *Controversies in Caring for Women with Epilepsy*, DOI 10.1007/978-3-319-29170-3_13

Author #1's Response

I would acknowledge her valid concerns regarding treatment with antiepileptic drugs (AEDs) during pregnancy, and will proceed as follows.

There are fetal/maternal risks related to AED during pregnancy which will be discussed including teratogenesis (anatomic defects and effects on the neurodevelopment) in the offspring.

Before counselling, following details are needed.

- Medical History: Past history including general health, psychiatric comorbidities, history of cardiac or significant other system involvement.
- Personal History: smoking, drug/alcohol use, educational/job status, ancestry.
- Medication History: Chronic medication use, use of folic acid.
- Family History: epilepsy, neural tube defects.
- Epilepsy History: Aura before seizure, history of spells with unresponsiveness, early morning myoclonus, focal features with seizure. Details regarding ER visit—electrolytes, BP, toxicology screen.

With the above information, EEG/MRI reports we can conclude that the patient has new onset epilepsy with generalized seizures. The presence of left temporal spikes suggests that the seizure likely has focal onset and NOT Genetic Generalized Epilepsy.

Counselling for AED Treatment

Treatment with an AED is necessary because the risk of additional seizures is very high. Patients with epilepsy can be at risk for uncontrolled seizures and status epilepticus, although risk of these events during pregnancy is not clear [1]. Seizure-related accidents can cause physical injuries to the mother and fetus. GTCS can cause alterations in electrolytes, blood pressure, and oxygenation, which can be detrimental to the immature brain. Recurrent GTCS during pregnancy has been found to affect neurodevelopment in some studies but not clearly proven. It has been noted that even when the cognitive abilities are not affected, convulsive seizure exposure can lead to increased educational needs in the child [2]. Increased mortality related to epilepsy can occur as with an epilepsy patient, including accidental death, sudden unexpected death in epilepsy [SUDEP], death from status epilepticus, suicides, complications of AED, but whether pregnancy confers increased mortality is not clear. The presence of GTCS and nocturnal seizures are risk factors for SUDEP [3] in this patient.

AED Choices

Carbamazepine (CBZ), lamotrigine (LTG), and levetiracetam (LEV) are possible treatment options.

Concern Regarding AED Use in Pregnancy

Maternal complications include idiosyncratic/acute adverse events due to new treatment with AED. There is a small risk of suicidal ideation or depression on AEDs. AED levels can change rapidly and need close monitoring during pregnancy and delivery to avoid toxicity and subtherapeutic levels.

Neonates exposed to AED in utero are probably at increased risk for being small for gestational age and possibly at increased risk of 1-min Apgar scores of <7. With CBZ and LTG exposure in utero, the rate of major congenital malformations (MCMs) (cardiac defects, cleft, etc.) may be at most twofold higher than expected [4]. The evidence so far indicates that in-utero exposure to CBZ or LTG is not associated with poorer neurodevelopment [2, 5, 6] although relationship between CBZ use and reduced verbal abilities needs further exploration. Data pertaining to the cognitive abilities of older children exposed to LTG are limited [2, 5]. As for LEV, malformation risk does not appear to be increased from the background rate, however there is lack of evidence regarding neurodevelopmental outcome with the use of LEV in pregnant women [5].

VPA should be avoided due to poorer cognitive outcome (7–10 IQ point reduction) in children exposed to VPA in utero [2, 5, 6] when compared to children exposed to other AEDs or controls. Furthermore children exposed to VPA have an increased risk of autistic spectrum disorders [5] and a higher prevalence of MCMs (from 4.7 to 13.8 %) with a dose-dependent effect [4].

AED Treatment of Choice

Considering all these, CBZ may be a good choice for this patient. LTG, although an option, cannot be up titrated quickly and that would place the women at risk for more seizures during the titration period. LEV albeit attractive, has very limited data regarding fetal safety. Monotherapy with lowest effective dose will be the best therapeutic strategy. Depending upon the ancestry, genetic testing for HLA-B*1502 is recommended before initiation of CBZ therapy [7].

She should be informed that AED treatment is a joint decision making. CBZ has been recommended, but if she chose to use LEV, her decision should be supported, as long as she understands the reasoning behind these choices.

Role of periconceptual folate on cognitive development needs further clarification due to conflicting results from existing studies [2, 6].

If she is a smoker, she should stop smoking, as smoking during pregnancy has an increased risk of premature contractions, premature labor and delivery. Alcohol can be a teratogen and should be avoided. Seizure precautions and precipitants should be discussed.

The women should be informed that there is uncertainty both to our current knowledge and to what these risks mean to the individual. This information can be overwhelming for the patient. Social work consult to provide emotional support can be helpful.

It is important to inform the patient that most women with epilepsy have healthy babies. It has been noted that cognitive outcome of children exposed to AED continue to improve with age [6]. At-risk children are targeted for closer developmental monitoring and get early intervention as indicated.

Author #2's Response

Witnessed, generalized tonic-clonic activity from sleep associated with tongue biting is highly suggestive of a seizure. Two unprovoked seizures >24 h apart is suggestive of a diagnosis of epilepsy. The presence of epileptiform discharges on EEG supports clinical diagnosis of likely a focal onset seizure with secondary generalization. In the context of normal exam and normal imaging, lack of triggers or prodromal illnesses, it is unlikely that the seizures are provoked by an acute pathology in this patient, such as infection, inflammation, sinus thrombosis, ischemia, or trauma. The preeclampsia is also unlikely in the first trimester pregnancy. Although only one-third will have recurrence after the first unprovoked seizure, the recurrence rate is 73 % within 4 years after two unprovoked seizures, highest occurrence being in the first year [8]. With the abnormal EEG, the treatment may be justified even after the first unprovoked seizure. There is also higher risk of worsening seizures in the second and third trimester pregnancy with a first trimester seizure [9]. Thus the patient should be offered an AED therapy for prevention of the breakthrough seizures.

The choice of AED should be based on patient age, comorbidities, type of epilepsy, and risks involved with the pregnancy. While most broad and narrow-spectrum AEDs are suitable as an initial choice for focal epilepsy, monotherapy in the lowest dose that controls the breakthrough seizures is the ideal goal to reduce the risks of MCMs in a pregnant woman. The MCM are 1–2 % in general population, and about 2.5× higher in women with epilepsy. Some common malformations include neural tube defects, cardiovascular anomalies, hypospadias, and oral clefts [9, 10]. Lamotrigine ($\approx$2 % risk of MCM), levetiracetam ($\approx$2.4 % risk of MCM) or carbamazepine ($\approx$2.9 % risk of MCM) showed better dose-dependent profile across all pregnancy registries [9–11]. The lamotrigine at 400 mg and carbamazepine at or <600 mg were associated with the least risk of major malformations [10]. Levetiracetam has an advantage of faster titration and more steady serum-levels, whereas longer titration and closer serum level monitoring is needed with lamotrigine. Newer generation AED has an advantage of lesser drug–drug interactions, lesser enzyme-inducing properties, and reduced risk of osteoporosis. The valproic acid should be avoided as it carries the highest risk of MCM and impaired neurodevelopmental outcomes in children exposed to Valproate in utero, and followed up to 6 years of age in comparison to other AED [6]. Phenobarbital ideally also is to be avoided due to higher risk of malformations [10]. Serum drug levels should be monitored monthly.

The patient will be counseled that there is high risk for injury, falls, and unexplained death in uncontrolled epilepsy. Generalized tonic-clonic seizures during pregnancy may cause maternal and fetal hypoxia, fetal heart-rate decelerations, miscarriages, stillbirths, rupture of membranes resulting in increased risk of infection, and premature labor. The patient should be educated and reassured. Despite the risks, most children are born healthy from pregnant women with epilepsy especially on monotherapy. The most fetal organ-development occurs within the first few weeks. In this woman, risks of fetal malformations may be even lower as there was no AED exposure during conception. A fetal ultrasound at 18 weeks should be performed. Folate supplementation to be continued [12]. Encourage avoiding sleep deprivation, excessive stress, and compliance. Future discussions should involve breastfeeding; sleep hygiene and safe caring for the child in postpartum period.

Reviewer's Comments

Both Author #1 and Author #2 are in agreement that the presented pregnant patient should be offered to start on anticonvulsant therapy due to high risk for seizure recurrence in her. They both argue the potential harm to the fetus as a result of maternal seizures including but not limited to falls and injury, maternal and fetal hypoxia, fetal heart-rate decelerations, miscarriages, stillbirths, and rupture of membranes resulting in increased risk of premature labor and infection. Therefore the authors both advocate starting the patient on seizure medication.

The choice of therapy as the authors point out is limited by potential for teratogenic side effects of the medications. In North American AED Pregnancy Registry (NAAPR), lamotrigine monotherapy during pregnancy was associated with a 2 % risk of malformation in the fetus. Carbamazepine monotherapy carried a risk of 3.0 %, phenytoin 2.9 %, topiramate 4.2 %, phenobarbital 6.5 %, and valproic acid 10.7 % in the offspring of women with epilepsy. The data for levetiracetam, oxcarbazepine, and gabapentin is limited but so far does not appear to show increased risk to the fetus from existing background risk (levetiracetam (2.4 %), oxcarbazepine (2.2 %) gabapentin (0.7 %)). The authors both give consideration to three choices namely carbamazepine, lamotrigine, and levetiracetam for more favorable side-effect profile during pregnancy based on the available data from multiple pregnancy registries. They both agree that despite low risk for MCM with lamotrigine, the prolonged titration period discourages starting the already pregnant patient on the medication. That will leave the choice of carbamazepine or levetiracetam more attractive.

Further, monitoring of AED levels during pregnancy is recommended [13]. Levels of carbamazepine are very stable during pregnancy, with a variability of only 10–12 %. This may provide an advantage over lamotrigine, for which clearance may increase up to 300 % in the second and third trimester. Therefore, the feasibility of following levels during pregnancy may be a factor in AED choice as well.

In summary, based on available data, there is a general agreement of practitioners in the field of epilepsy that it is likely more safe to start women with new onset epilepsy on seizure medication during their pregnancy. The reasonable choices for partial onset epilepsy in pregnant women based on the currently available data are carbamazepine, lamotrigine, and levetiracetam. Practitioners may take the ease and safety of titration and patient's choice into account when recommending starting a pregnant patient with new onset epilepsy on medication.

Suggested Management

1. For a pregnant patient with newly diagnosed partial onset epilepsy, current evidence supports starting on anticonvulsant therapy.
2. When counselling the pregnant patient explain the potential risks of seizures to her and her fetus and how the benefits of seizure control by certain medications may outweigh the potentially teratogenic side effects.
3. Consider carbamazepine, oxcarbazepine, lamotrigine, and levetiracetam as choices of therapy in a pregnant woman with newly diagnosed epilepsy.
4. Ease of titration and patient's risk for seizure recurrence should be taken into account when recommending the above anticonvulsant medications to pregnant women.
5. Availability of therapeutic drug monitoring and in that light, stability of AED levels over the course of the pregnancy is also a consideration in AED choice.

References

1. Harden CL, Hopp J, Ting TY, Pennell PB, French JA, Hauser WA, et al. Practice parameter update: management issues for women with epilepsy—focus on pregnancy (an evidence-based review): obstetrical complications and change in seizure frequency: report of the Quality Standards Subcommittee and Therapeutics and Technology Assessment Subcommittee of the American Academy of Neurology and American Epilepsy Society. Neurology. 2009;73(2):126–32.
2. Baker GA, Bromley RL, Briggs M, Cheyne CP, Cohen MJ, Garcia-Finana M, et al. IQ at 6 years after in utero exposure to antiepileptic drugs: a controlled cohort study. Neurology. 2015;84(4):382–90.
3. Hesdorffer DC, Tomson T. Sudden unexpected death in epilepsy. Potential role of antiepileptic drugs. CNS Drugs. 2013;27(2):113–9.
4. Tomson T, Xue H, Battino D. Major congenital malformations in children of women with epilepsy. Seizure. 2015;28:46–50.
5. Bromley R, Weston J, Adab N, Greenhalgh J, Sanniti A, McKay AJ, et al. Treatment for epilepsy in pregnancy: neurodevelopment outcomes in the child. Cochrane Database Syst Rev. 2014;10:CD010236.
6. Meador KJ, Baker GA, Browning N, Cohen MJ, Bromley RL, Clayton-Smith J, et al. Fetal antiepileptic drug exposure and cognitive outcomes at age 6 years (NEAD study): a prospective observational study. Lancet Neurol. 2013;12(3):244–52.
7. Amstutz U, Shear NH, Rieder MJ, Hwang S, Fung V, Nakamura H, et al. Recommendations for HLA-B*15:02 and HLA-A*31:01 genetic testing to reduce the risk of carbamazepine-induced hypersensitivity reactions. Epilepsia. 2014;55(4):496–506.
8. Hauser WA, Rich SS, et al. Risk of recurrent seizures after two unprovoked seizures. N Engl J Med. 1998;338:429–34.
9. Battino D, Tomson T, Bonizzoni E, Craig J, et al. Seizure control and treatment changes in pregnancy: observations from the EURAP epilepsy pregnancy registry. Epilepsia. 2013;54(9):1621–7.

10. Hernández-Díaz S, Smith CR, Shen A, Mittendorf R, et al. Comparative safety of antiepileptic drugs during pregnancy. Neurology. 2012;78:1692–9.
11. Schmidt D, Schachter S. Drug treatment of epilepsy in adults. BMJ. 2014;348:g2456.
12. Harden C, et al. Management issues for women with epilepsy—focus on pregnancy (an evidence-based review): II. Teratogenesis and perinatal outcomes. Epilepsia. 2009;50(5):1237–46.
13. Harden CL, Pennell PB, Koppel BS, Hovinga CA, Gidal B, Meador KJ, Hopp J, Ting TY, Hauser WA, Thurman D, Kaplan PW, Robinson JN, French JA, Wiebe S, Wilner AN, Vazquez B, Holmes L, Krumholz A, Finnell R, Shafer PO, Le Guen C, American Academy of Neurology, American Epilepsy Society. Practice parameter update: management issues for women with epilepsy—focus on pregnancy (an evidence-based review): vitamin K, folic acid, blood levels, and breastfeeding: report of the Quality Standards Subcommittee and Therapeutics and Technology Assessment Subcommittee of the American Academy of Neurology and American Epilepsy Society. Neurology. 2009;73(2):142–9.

Chapter 14
Valproic Acid and Pregnancy

Jakob Christensen and Sean Tchanho Hwang

Case Scenario

A 26-year-old woman (G2P1) is referred to you for consultation. She is in her second month of pregnancy and on valproic acid 1000 mg twice daily for her medically stable Juvenile Myoclonic Epilepsy. She has not had any seizure recurrences in the past year. Would you lower valproic acid; discontinue it or switch to another seizure medication during her current pregnancy? If you would switch her seizure medication, what would you switch to and how do you manage her epilepsy during this pregnancy?

Author #1's Response

Valproic acid in monotherapy is effective for idiopathic generalized epilepsy (including Juvenile Myoclonic Epilepsy) [1]. However, valproic acid, when used in pregnancy, is associated with dose-dependent risks of major congenital malformations (MCMs) and reduction in cognitive abilities in the offspring [2]. Therefore,

J. Christensen, Ph.D., M.D.
Department of Neurology, Aarhus University Hospital,
Noerrebrogade 44, Aarhus, Denmark 8000
e-mail: jakob@farm.au.dk

S.T. Hwang, M.D.
Department of Neurology, North Shore University Hospital, Hofstra North Shore LIJ Comprehensive Epilepsy Care Center, 611 Northern Boulevard, Suite 150, Great Neck, NY 11021, USA
e-mail: shwang2@nshs.edu

Commentator: C.L. Harden, M.D. (✉)
Mount Sinai Health System, Mount Sinai Beth Israel Phillips Ambulatory Care Center, 10 Union Square East, Suite 5D, New York, NY 10003, USA
e-mail: charden@chpnet.org

© Springer International Publishing Switzerland 2016
M. Sazgar, C.L. Harden (eds.), *Controversies in Caring for Women with Epilepsy*, DOI 10.1007/978-3-319-29170-3_14

both the European Medicines Agency and the U.S. Food and Drug Administration warn that valproic acid should be used in pregnant women with epilepsy only if other treatments have failed to provide adequate seizure control or are otherwise unaccept-able—ideally a decision to stop treatment with valproic acid should be made prior to pregnancy. Unfortunately, a significant proportion of pregnancies are unplanned—e.g., in the United States, nearly half (49 %) of the 6.4 million pregnancies each year are unintended—this proportion is likely of a similar size in women with epilepsy. Given the effectiveness of valproic acid in Juvenile Myoclonic Epilepsy, it is likely that also in the future, a number of fertile women will end up in a situation where they must consider continuous treatment with valproic acid during pregnancy.

At this early stage of pregnancy (second month), there are a number of treatment options that the pregnant woman will likely discuss with her treating physician. Firstly, the physician will be able to inform her that at this time of pregnancy most of the fetal organs have already been formed (Fig. 14.1), and for that reason, it is too late to alter treatment in order to reduce the risk of MCMs such as spina bifida because the neural tube closes about 1 month after conception. So if the woman is still taking valproic acid at the time when she realizes that she is pregnant (usually after a missed period in the second month of pregnancy), it is often recommended that she continue treatment with valproic acid throughout pregnancy [3]. However, the internal organs including the heart and not least the brain continue to develop throughout pregnancy and thus continuous treatment with valproic acid will still be a matter of concern [2].

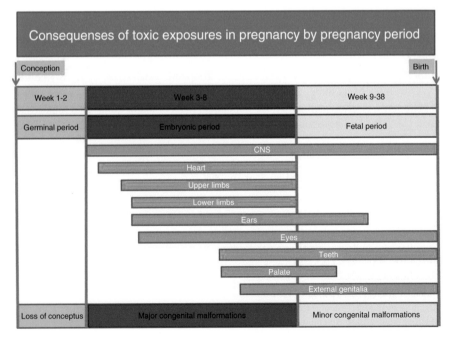

Fig. 14.1 Consequences of toxic exposures in pregnancy by pregnancy period

Discontinuation or Tapering of Valproic Acid

Abrupt discontinuation of valproic acid (or any other antiepileptic drug [AED]) poses a risk of seizure recurrence including status epilepticus and even occasionally death and is therefore not advisable although, sometimes chosen by pregnant women without consulting her physician. Gradual tapering of the valproic acid dose would be an option often discussed, but Juvenile Myoclonic Epilepsy carries a high risk of seizure recurrence after medication withdrawal. Lower doses of valproic acid during pregnancy is associated with lower risk of congenital malformation and adverse cognitive development [4]; but it has never been shown that women on an initial high dose (i.e. >1000 mg/ day) who reduce the daily dose of valproic acid will also be able to reduce the risk associated with valproic acid in pregnancy. Therefore, switching to another AED with lower risk would be an option, but again, there is little evidence to support that switching from valproic acid to another AED will result in improved development of the fetus.

Switching to Another AED

Should the woman—after consultation with her physician—choose to change AED during pregnancy, then the treatment options for a patient with Juvenile Myoclonic Epilepsy will usually include lamotrigine, levetiracetam, and topiramate.

Based on results from pregnancy registers, the lowest risk of congenital malformations and adverse cognitive development is found following pregnancies with lamotrigine [4]. However, the transition from valproic acid to lamotrigine monotherapy is complex and slow (Table 14.1)—especially during pregnancy. In this situation, the metabolism of lamotrigine is influenced by both an inhibited metabolism by concomitant valproic acid therapy as well as an increased excretion of lamotrigine induced by the pregnancy. These factors require frequent dose adjustments—often guided by monthly plasma level measurements. In addition, lamotrigine may be less effective than valproic acid in Juvenile Myoclonic Epilepsy [1]—especially against myoclonic seizures. In the case or reemerging myoclonic seizures—a small dose of clonazepam (1–2 mg daily) may often be sufficient to alleviate myoclonic seizures. However, this approach has not been subject to systematic studies or approval.

Topiramate is another treatment alternative for Juvenile Myoclonic Epilepsy [1]. However, experience in pregnancy with this drug is limited and preliminary results seem to suggest that topiramate is associated with both an increased risk of congenital malformations [3] as well as an increased risk of intrauterine growth restriction [5]. Thus, switching from valproic acid to topiramate is not advisable with the current knowledge of the risks associated with the two drugs [3].

Levetiracetam is an AED that is effective against Juvenile Myoclonic Epilepsy, although the efficacy may not be as good as with valproic acid. The titration to a relevant therapeutic dose is relatively quick (Table 14.1), but the experience with

Table 14.1 Rapid transition from valproic acid monotherapy to alternative lamotrigine, topiramate, and levetiracetam monotherapy for the treatment of juvenile myoclonic epilepsy in pregnancy

AED	Daily dosing[a]	Week 1	2	3	4	5	6	7	8
Valproic acid	Morning dose	1000	1000	500	0				
	Evening dose	1000	500	500	0				
Levetiracetam	Morning dose	250	500						
	Evening dose	250	500						
Topiramate	Morning dose	25	25	50	75	100			
	Evening dose	0	25	50	75	100			
Lamotrigine[b]	Morning dose	12.5[c]	12.5[c]	25	25	25	50	100	
	Evening dose	0	0	0	0	25	50	100	

[a]Daily dosing may be divided into three, if not thought to compromise compliance
[b]Lamotrigine dose should be further adjusted according to clinical efficacy/side effects. Lamotrigine treatment may be guided by plasma level measurements to account for interactions with valproic acid and increased metabolism of lamotrigine during pregnancy
[c]25 mg taken every other day

levetiracetam in pregnancy is limited. The evidence—so far—is not suggestive of an increased malformation risk [3], but the potential effects on cognitive development as well as neuropsychiatric disorders such as autism is currently not established.

In conclusion: all fertile women should receive counselling of the risks associated with epilepsy and AED treatment during pregnancy. This counselling should ideally take place prior to pregnancy in order to fully discuss treatment alternatives, adjust AED type, dose and dosing schedule as well as ensuring folic acid supplementation. Regular visits or contacts during pregnancy, e.g., once monthly will help ensure best possible treatment as well as ensure optimal compliance.

Author #2's Response

Few scenarios in the care of women with epilepsy may be as anxiety provoking as the pronouncement of one's patient that she is pregnant while taking valproic acid (VPA). The physician experiences a sinking feeling in inverse proportion to the mounting evidence that has accumulated in regards to the deleterious effects of this drug on fetal development. Several databases analyzing the outcome of pregnancies of patients on AEDs have had one consistent finding in that VPA appears to the most harmful. In monotherapy, the rate of MCMs has been reported to be near 9.3–9.7 % [4, 6]. The risk appears to be dose related with MCMs occurring at a considerably

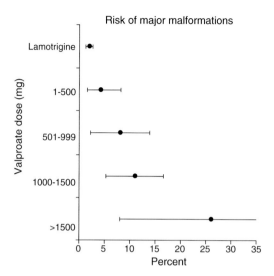

Fig. 14.2 Risk of major malformations by average valproate dose (mg) during the first trimester (From Hernández-Díaz S, Smith CR, Shen A, Mittendorf R, Hauser WA, Yerby M, Holmes LB. North American AED Pregnancy Registry. Comparative safety of antiepileptic drugs during pregnancy. Neurology. 2012 May 22;78(21):1692–9 with permission)

higher rate with exposures over 1000 mg per day [6]. The EURAP international study group found the risk of MCMs to be 4.2 % at exposures under 700 mg/day, 9.0 % between 700 and 1500 mg per day, and up to 23.2 % at doses at or above 1500 mg per day [4]. A wide range of MCMs have been described including neural tube, cardiac, orofacial, genitourinary, and skeletal abnormalities (Fig. 14.2).

A recent prospective longitudinal cohort study has also demonstrated long-term negative effects of intrauterine VPA exposure on cognitive development in children assessed at 6 years of age [7]. With maternal VPA doses above 800 mg per day, children had an adjusted mean reduction in IQ of 9.7 points; with significant deficits in verbal, nonverbal, and spatial abilities in comparison to control children and those exposed to lamotrigine or carbamazepine. The risk of IQ reduction was mitigated by doses of VPA below 800 mg; yet, these children still had higher rates of verbal impairments and greater needs for educational intervention. A higher overall incidence of autism spectrum disorder in children exposed to VPA was also described (Fig. 14.3).

Our patient has presented in her first trimester, but past the gestational age of neural tube closure, and it remains possible that major deformity cannot be averted. Nonetheless, the precise effects of the timing of when exposure to VPA occurs in relation to gestational age on fetal development remains unclear, particularly in regards to long-term cognitive outcomes. Therefore, reduction or cessation of VPA, or a substitution with an alternate AED may still be important considerations.

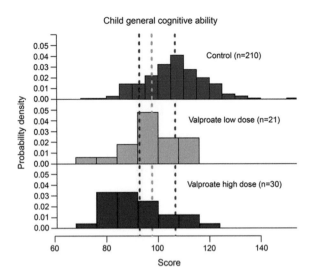

Fig. 14.3 Distribution of IQ scores across the control and valproate-exposed groups (From Baker GA, Bromley RL, Briggs M, Cheyne CP, Cohen MJ, García-Fiñana M, Gummery A, Kneen R, Loring DW, Mawer G, Meador KJ, Shallcross R, Clayton-Smith J. IQ at 6 years after in utero exposure to antiepileptic drugs: A controlled cohort study. Neurology. 2015 Jan 27;84(4):382–90 with permission)

After a careful interview to understand the historical response of her seizures to VPA dose escalation, one might advocate lowering the dose of VPA if adequate seizure control is maintained and if the patient is willing to accept some level of associated risk. Frequent myoclonus or staring spells would be a serious red flag to reinitiate therapy at higher doses, should they occur. To understand the patient's baseline degree of seizure control, a baseline video-EEG could be helpful, to assess for spike abundance or subtle clinical myoclonus or absence. A follow-up video-EEG may likewise offer information about abnormal cortical activity or subtle clinical events subsequent to medication reduction. Lower VPA doses have been associated with a lower risk of MCM, and theoretically, divided doses or extended release versions of the drug may further decrease maximal peak concentrations.

A less appealing approach, particularly in the early weeks of pregnancy, would be to proceed with medication cessation. The obvious risk to the patient and the developing fetus would involve the recurrence of seizures carrying the risk of personal injury, SUDEP, accidents, loss of independence for the patient, and possible deleterious effects on the fetus. Discontinuation of AED therapy would certainly necessitate careful discussion with the patient and others involved with her care regarding the relative risks and benefits of doing so, the restriction of driving, and having measures in place for clinical support and emergency medications should seizures occur.

We know in our patient's case that overt seizures have not occurred within the last year. While we generally consider JME to confer a lifelong risk of seizure recurrence with a high rate of relapse, a few patients may have relatively infrequent seizures or long stretches devoid of debilitating seizures, even with discontinuation of medication. A recent longitudinal study of the long-term prognosis of patients with JME did in fact indicate 16.7 % of patients eventually remaining seizure free off medication for greater than 5 years [8]. Absence seizures appear to be a negative predictor of seizure remission. If our patient's seizures have been historically very infrequent, and have not occurred in many years, perhaps one might be tempted to consider reduction or cessation of medication, at least until the later trimesters. The risk of breakthrough convulsions occurring during early pregnancy would be the main deterrent.

The last consideration would be transition to an alternate AED. Given her syndrome, one would prudently select from a broader spectrum AED such as levetiracetam, topiramate, zonisamide, or lamotrigine. Lamotrigine has one of the most favorable teratogenicity profiles in the treatment of pregnant women with epilepsy. The North American AED Pregnancy Registry found rates of malformation of 2.4 % [6]. Primarily a sodium channel blocker, it has been approved for use in patients with idiopathic generalized epilepsy, but maybe associated with exacerbation of myoclonus. In addition, the slow titration required due to the risk of dermatological reactions, the need for cross over polytherapy, and the effects on drug levels due to pregnancy and interactions with VPA would likely make this choice impractical. Topiramate and zonisamide are efficacious in the care of patients with JME, and are probably of intermediate teratogenic risk. Topiramate is associated with a risk of cleft lip and had an overall risk of MCM near 4.2 %. Less data is available for the use of zonisamide. Levetiracetam (LEV), on the other hand, is considered a broad spectrum AED with good overall tolerability and low risk for serious systemic adverse reactions. LEV may be one of the safer AEDs available in the treatment of pregnant women with epilepsy with rates of MCM near 2.4 % in monotherapy [6]. Though any transition would preferably be done prior to pregnancy, rapid titration on LEV is typically well-tolerated, and conversion from VPA could be done in a relatively swift manner. Emerging data supports the efficacy of LEV as an alternative first-line agent in JME [9]. LEV has been useful in patients with poor tolerability to VPA, though comparative data evaluating its efficacy versus VPA in JME is lacking.

The final decision would take into deliberation the patient's historical seizure frequency, prior experience with other AEDs, reliability, mood stability, fear of seizures, adversity to risk, willingness to abstain from driving, and our shared concerns for the health of the fetus. As the patient remains in the first trimester where some benefit of a substitution may be realized, if in alignment with the patient's own wishes, recommendations would be for a rapid transition to an intermediate dose of LEV in extended release form and cessation of VPA. Preferably this would be performed in a setting such as the epilepsy monitoring unit with baseline extended EEG recording, then with subsequent outpatient EEG recording in the following month. Though this approach may have some risk of seizure breakthrough, the data increasingly suggests that there may ultimately be no safe therapeutic dose of VPA. I would recommend extra precautions be taken in regards to seizure safety, and cessation of driving at least for the short-term while medications are being adjusted. Should seizures recur, dose escalation may be required, or a transition back to VPA at lower doses in extended release form as tolerated, with adjunctive treatment if necessary, particularly if later in gestation. The patient would be asked to continue with prenatal vitamin and folic acid supplementation, as well as close obstetrical follow-up.

Reviewer's Comments

In this case scenario, probably one of the most challenging of this book, author #2 eloquently expresses the feelings of dread on the part of the treating physician evoked by this situation. Both authors discuss the high rates of teratogenesis expected at the valproate dose used, and that major organogenesis has already taken place. In other words, it's too late to prevent MCMs. What to do now is presented in detail by both authors, and includes lowering the dose, changing AEDs with levetiracetam presented as an option, but neither author advocated stopping the drug at this point during pregnancy. Author #2 emphasized the use of the epilepsy monitoring unit for ongoing evaluation as medications are adjusted. There were also some lifestyle interventions, such as asking her to stop driving during the time of medication alteration.

But getting back to the "sinking feeling," discussed by Author #2, we should think about really why would this occur? It occurs not only for concern regarding the developing fetus, but secondarily and overwhelmingly, it occurs because one wonders if everything was done to try to change from valproate to a safer option in the 26-year-old woman before she was pregnant, or if appropriate guidance was provided regarding contraception.

It is not stated in this vignette whether the pregnancy was planned or unplanned. Try as we might, we cannot completely prevent unplanned pregnancies; is beyond our purview of care to control personal behavior. But it would decrease the "sinking feeling" if it was clearly documented that other AEDs were tried in this 26-year-old woman, leaving valproate as the best option. In this case the valproate dose should be minimized hopefully to less than 700 mg per day, the dose at which the rate of MCMs appears to be mostly below threshold for the adverse effect [10]. The discussion regarding birth control should be documented and hand-in-hand with this, the discussion in which the patient is informed and appears to understand the risks of getting pregnant while taking valproate should be documented, which is AAN quality measure #6 [11].

As care providers, we usually cannot stop our patients from getting pregnant, and we cannot reverse the risk that has already taken place due to first trimester exposure. But we can change the cause of the "sinking feeling" by adherence to current recommendations for avoiding valproate use in women of childbearing potential [3], and by regular discussion of contraception, and of course, documentation of such.

Suggested Management

In case of a pregnant woman who is already taking valproate:

1. Obtain detailed information about the patient's response to valproate and consider reducing dose.
2. Consider changing to another AED such as levetiracetam under inpatient observation and/or continuous video-EEG monitoring.
3. Implement checklists into your EMR to make sure pregnancy risks and contraception are discussed and women of childbearing age are on daily folic acid supplement.

References

1. Marson AG, Al-Kharusi AM, Alwaidh M, Appleton R, Baker GA, Chadwick DW, et al. The SANAD study of effectiveness of valproate, lamotrigine, or topiramate for generalized and unclassifiable epilepsy: an unblended randomized controlled trial. Lancet. 2007;369(9566):1016–26.
2. Meador KJ, Baker GA, Browning N, Cohen MJ, Bromley RL, Clayton-Smith J, et al. Fetal antiepileptic drug exposure and cognitive outcomes at age 6 years (NEAD study): a prospective observational study. Lancet Neurol. 2013;12(3):244–52.
3. Tomson T, Marson A, Boon P, Canevini MP, Covanis A, Gaily E, et al. Valproate in the treatment of epilepsy in women and girls Recommendations from a joint Task Force of ILAE-Commission on European Affairs and European Academy of Neurology (EAN). Epilepsia. 2015;8:10.
4. Tomson T, Battino D, Bonizzoni E, Craig J, Lindhout D, Sabers A, et al. Dose-dependent risk of malformations with antiepileptic drugs: an analysis of data from the EURAP epilepsy and pregnancy registry. Lancet Neurol. 2011;10(7):609–17.
5. Kilic D, Pedersen H, Kjaersgaard MI, Parner ET, Vestergaard M, Sorensen MJ, et al. Birth outcomes after prenatal exposure to antiepileptic drugs—a population-based study. Epilepsia. 2014;55(11):1714–21.
6. Hernández-Díaz S, Smith CR, Shen A, Mittendorf R, Hauser WA, Yerby M, Holmes LB, North American AED Pregnancy Registry. Comparative safety of antiepileptic drugs during pregnancy. Neurology. 2012;78(21):1692–9.
7. Baker GA, Bromley RL, Briggs M, Cheyne CP, Cohen MJ, García-Fiñana M, Gummery A, Kneen R, Loring DW, Mawer G, Meador KJ, Shallcross R, Clayton-Smith J. IQ at 6 years after in utero exposure to antiepileptic drugs: a controlled cohort study. Neurology. 2015;84(4):382–90.
8. Senf P, Schmitz B, Holtkamp M, Janz D. Prognosis of juvenile myoclonic epilepsy 45 years after onset: seizure outcome and predictors. Neurology. 2013;81(24):2128–33.
9. Crespel A, Gelisse P, Reed RC, Ferlazzo E, Jerney J, Schmitz B, Genton P. Management of juvenile myoclonic epilepsy. Epilepsy Behav. 2013;28 Suppl 1:S81–6.
10. Tomson T, Battino D, Bonizzoni E, Craig J, Lindhout D, Perucca E, Sabers A, Thomas SV, Vajda F, EURAP Study Group. Dose-dependent teratogenicity of valproate in mono- and polytherapy: an observational study. Neurology. 2015;85(10):866–72.
11. Fountain NB, Van Ness PC, Bennett A, Absher J, Patel AD, Sheth KN, Gloss DS, Morita DA, Stecker M. Quality improvement in neurology: epilepsy update quality measurement set. Neurology. 2015;84(14):1483–7.

Chapter 15
Lamotrigine and Pregnancy

Jennifer L. Hopp and David G. Vossler

Case Scenario

A 29-year-old woman is followed by you as her epileptologist for the past 5 years. She has a diagnosis of focal epilepsy of right lateral temporal lobe origin due to cortical dysplasia. She is on lamotrigine 100 mg twice daily and was seizure free for 2 years. She makes an urgent appointment with you due to experiencing a generalized tonic-clonic seizure while teaching in her classroom. When at your office she informs you that she is 5 weeks pregnant. On further questioning, she has experienced three episodes of auras in the past 2 weeks. She is wondering whether she has to increase the dose of lamotrigine. She has several questions including how often she needs to be checked for the lamotrigine levels and how much does she need to increase the dose by. She is worried and is asking you whether the increase in the dose of lamotrigine will increase the risk to her baby. How do you manage lowering the lamotrigine dose in the immediate postpartum period and thereafter?

J.L. Hopp, M.D.
Department of Neurology, University of Maryland School of Medicine,
Maryland Epilepsy Center, 22 S. Greene St. S12C09, Baltimore, MD 21201, USA
e-mail: jhopp@som.umaryland.edu

D.G. Vossler, M.D., F.A.A.N.
Valley Medical Center, Neuroscience Institute, University of Washington,
400 South 43rd Street, Renton, WA 98055, USA
e-mail: dgvossler@msn.com

Commentator: M. Sazgar, M.D. (✉)
University of California, Irvine Medical Center,
101 The City Drive South, Pavilion I, Bldg. 30, Suite 123, Orange, CA 92868, USA
e-mail: msazgar@uci.edu

© Springer International Publishing Switzerland 2016
M. Sazgar, C.L. Harden (eds.), *Controversies in Caring for Women with Epilepsy*, DOI 10.1007/978-3-319-29170-3_15

Author #1's Response

Our patient is a young woman who recently experienced a generalized tonic-clonic seizure while taking lamotrigine 100 mg twice daily. She has a malformation of cortical development (which is likely responsible for her temporal lobe epilepsy), had been seizure free for 2 years prior to this recent convulsion, and now finds herself in the first trimester of pregnancy. This case presents several management concerns which will need to be addressed at the present, over the next 9 months, and while breastfeeding. The questions to be addressed are the case for and against the use of antiepileptic drugs (AEDs) during pregnancy, including the rates of adverse effects of different AEDs used during pregnancy, and the pharmacokinetics of lamotrigine during and after pregnancy.

The case for and against the use of AEDs during pregnancy can be conceptualized as being related to three issues: the risk of injury and death to mother and fetus, the chance of teratogenesis, and the risk of neurodevelopmental effects in the offspring. Most women who unexpectedly find themselves pregnant will ask their providers whether it is advisable to discontinue their AEDs, because they are at least somewhat aware of the elevated risk of birth malformations in their offspring. They often have a limited understanding of the dangers that seizures pose to the fetus and mother. It is the responsibility of the neurologist to guide patients to minimize both the risks that seizures cause during pregnancy as well as the risks that AEDs pose. Numerous studies have suggested that although non-convulsive seizures carry low risks of adverse effects on pregnancy, convulsive seizures can result in serious injuries and death. Generalized tonic-clonic seizures are associated with multiple adverse outcomes including: placental abruption, intracranial hemorrhage, miscarriage, stillbirth, fetal hypoxia and heart decelerations, and lower infant IQ. Status epilepticus carries the additional risk of maternal death. Most physicians feel that the risks of serious adverse effects of convulsive seizures outweigh the risks of AEDs. It is important that the provider have a gentle discussion with pregnant women with epilepsy (WWE) about these risks, ideally in advance of pregnancy.

Given the fact that our patient recently experienced a generalized tonic-clonic seizure, it is apparent that her 2 years of seizure freedom was not the result of the resolution of her epilepsy. For this reason, and because of the convulsive nature of the seizure, continued AED treatment is warranted. The next management decision is to choose an AED at a dose which not only likely will be effective but also carries a reasonably low risk of teratogenesis.

When considering the risks of AEDs in pregnancy, some research studies provide guidance. In the ongoing North American AED Pregnancy Registry (NAAEDPR), the risks of major fetal malformations have been calculated for many of the commonly used AEDs. Our patient is taking lamotrigine, and this is the AED which the greatest number of women in the NAAEDPR reported taking. As of this writing, the NAAEDPR has registered 1812 women who had taken lamotrigine monotherapy. Among them, the major malformation rate is 2.0 % (95 % confidence interval = 1.4–2.8 %). This compares favorably with the study's internal and external unexposed controls (1.2 % [0.46–2.7 %] and 1.6 % [1.5–1.7 %] respectively). The major malformation rate for lamotrigine is lower than the rates with certain other AEDs which might be considered for focal-onset epilepsies such as topiramate, phenobarbital, and valproate [1]. In a separate study, the International Lamotrigine Pregnancy Registry, the rate of major congenital malformations for monotherapy was similar at 2.2 % (95 % CI = 1.6–3.1 %) [2].

Although orofacial clefts were reported in high numbers with lamotrigine earlier in the course of the NAAEDPR study [3], other studies have not borne that out. Lamotrigine is known to have antifolate properties, which is one of the reasons it was tested in the U.S. National Institutes of Health AED development program. Because supplemental folic acid has been associated with a lower risk of cleft palate when given to healthy women, administration of folic acid has also been recommended for pregnant women taking lamotrigine. Prenatal vitamins generally contain 0.8 mg of folic acid, but we recommend an additional 2 mg of folic acid daily.

In addition to teratogenesis, one must consider the neurodevelopmental effects of AEDs on the fetus. Fewer studies inform our AED choice in this regard, but the best may be the Neurodevelopemental Effects of Antiepileptic Drugs (NEAD) study which recently published the 6-year follow-up developmental data on children exposed in utero to carbamazepine, lamotrigine, phenytoin, and valproate [4]. The NEAD study found at age 6 that children exposed in utero to lamotrigine, phenytoin, or carbamazepine had normal intelligence. Children exposed to lamotrigine had mean IQ at age 6 of 108 (CI = 105–110) compared to carbamazepine (105), phenytoin (108), and valproate (97). Verbal abilities were worse than nonverbal abilities in all groups, and in the lamotrigine and valproate groups.

Because lamotrigine is effective in focal-onset seizures, and has a favorable teratogenesis and neurodevelopmental profile, the next management decision is selecting the optimum dose for our patient. She is, like most women, hoping to take the minimum effective dose of lamotrigine. Based upon her recent generalized tonic-clonic seizure, an increase in her dose is indicated. Lamotrigine carries a low rate of producing very serious allergic skin reactions such as Stevens–Johnson syndrome or toxic epidermal necrolysis. Owing to this, the dose should not be increased from her current 100 mg BID dose at a rate of more than 50 mg/day at weekly intervals. This is prudent not only in patients who have been recently started on lamotrigine, but also in persons who have taken it for years. The dose approved by the U.S. Food and Drug Administration for monotherapy is 150 mg BID, but many experts would go higher depending on patient needs. Many experts use a lamotrigine serum level therapeutic range of 4–15 µg/mL. One needs to select an appropriate dose in the first and second trimesters, and check a trough serum level at that time. The reason is that serum lamotrigine levels have been reported to fall by 1/2–2/3 from the second to the third trimester. Pennell et al. described an increase of lamotrigine clearance of 94 % in the third trimester [5]. As a result, providers must monitor serum lamotrigine levels every 2–4 weeks during the third trimester, and increase the lamotrigine dose accordingly to maintain the first trimester level.

Beginning 2–3 weeks after delivery, it will be necessary to reduce the lamotrigine dose over about 2 weeks back down to the first trimester dose. If this is not done quickly enough, it is extremely common for the postpartum woman to complain of dizziness, blurred vision, diplopia, or ataxia.

Concerns are often raised by pediatricians about breastfeeding. When they counsel the new mother, they often inform the mother that starting an infant or child on lamotrigine has a much higher rate of serious cutaneous reaction than occurs with adults. However, serious rashes do not seem to occur in the children of WWE taking lamotrigine, presumably because the infant has been exposed to the drug throughout gestation. Concerns about neurodevelopmental effects from AED exposure in breast milk can be informed by the Norwegian Mother and Child Cohort Study [6]. Investigators in this study showed that continuous breastfeeding in the infants of women taking AEDs was associated with less impaired development at 6 and 18 months compared with those with no breastfeeding or breastfeeding for <6 months. Thus, we recommend breastfeeding by a woman taking lamotrigine, because the benefits to the woman seem to outweigh the risks.

Author #2's Response

The first principle to impart to women with regard to medication and seizure management during pregnancy is that most WWE do well during their pregnancies and most babies are born healthy. That said, there are several key points to discuss and there are special challenges when these discussions only occur after a woman reports her pregnancy. In addition, women who take lamotrigine for seizure control face unique issues that relate to the pharmacokinetics and clearance of this medication during their pregnancies. Further discussion is important to plan medication management as well as to review risks during the pregnancy to mother and baby. In addition to the questions to be addressed below, it is worthwhile having a comprehensive conversation about how to try to reduce risks of major malformations as well as how to keep her and her child safe with regard to seizure control during the pregnancy and after delivery.

Although pre-pregnancy planning may not be possible at this stage, hopefully she is already taking folate at a dose of at least 0.4 mg daily. Although the specific dose of folate used to prevent major malformations remains somewhat unclear, and the reduction in risk may be difficult to quantify, it is likely that taking folic acid in the preconception period may reduce risks of major malformations, so at 5 weeks gestation, this may still be worthwhile [7]. There may be other issues to discuss moving forward, but for the purposes of this exercise, let's focus on her questions first.

1. She is wondering whether she has to increase the dose of Lamotrigine.

It is important to increase the dose of lamotrigine for several reasons in this patient. First, she has just had a generalized tonic-clonic seizure (GTCS) after a relatively long seizure free period (of 2 years) as well as persistent auras with a history of focal-onset epilepsy. This suggests that her risk for recurrent seizures during the pregnancy may be higher than expected. In general, the fact that she was previously seizure free would be considered to be associated with a relatively high chance of remaining seizure free during the pregnancy [8], but her recent seizure suggests otherwise. It is important to explain that at least in a subset of WWE, the concentrations of lamotrigine may change significantly during pregnancy and in fact, a recent drop in the level (due to the drug being cleared more rapidly) may be the cause of her recent seizures. Data suggest that if she has had a drop in this concentration, it is likely to continue to occur, so a change in the dose is warranted [9]. If a pre-pregnancy level is available, a repeat level now is likely to show a decrease in the drug concentration. It is also important to emphasize that her history of GTCS could put her at risk for physical harm to the fetus due to falls or other injury.

2. She has several questions including how often she needs to be checked for the lamotrigine levels and how often might the dose be changed.

It is important here to explain that lamotrigine has relatively low risks for teratogenicity in her child [10], but at the same time, the concentration of the medication will likely reduce significantly during her pregnancy and may lead to further seizures or an increase in seizure frequency. Because it is difficult to know how much and how quickly these levels will drop due to individual variations, it's difficult to predict at this point how often we may need to draw levels. Hopefully, we will know more based on changes in the levels during the first trimester [9]. If we don't have a pre-pregnancy level, it is important to be checked now and to have levels done at least once a month through the first trimester [9]. After that time, we may be able to reduce checking the levels based on how much her levels drop (how much the clearance of the medication changes). The dose will be adjusted accordingly to try to maintain her first (or pre-pregnancy level) by achieving seizure control without adverse events [5].

3. She is worried and is asking you whether the increase in the dose of Lamotrigine will increase the risk to her baby.

It is unlikely that the increased dose of lamotrigine will increase the risk to her baby as the dose changes are needed to maintain her target drug concentration. It is possible that there are small changes in dose that are not necessary to maintain those levels but this may be difficult to quantify [9]. It's worthwhile reassuring her that the risks with lamotrigine during pregnancy are relatively low [10] and that these dose changes are needed to maintain a drug concentration to control her seizures. It's also worth discussing other risks such as risk to her fetus if she has seizures that lead to falls or other injuries and that the medication changes are being performed to mitigate that risk.

4. How do you manage lowering the Lamotrigine dose in the immediate postpartum period and thereafter?

It will be important to keep in touch following her pregnancy as changes may be needed in the first few weeks. Studies about the clearance of lamotrigine suggest that we may need to decrease and taper to her prepartum dose (or slightly higher if she had more seizures or is sensitive to sleep deprivation) within 3 weeks postpartum [9] (Fig. 15.1).

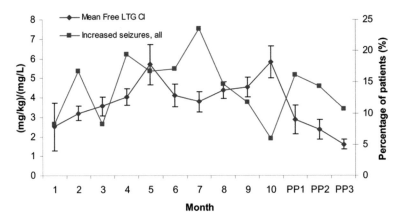

Fig. 15.1 Changes in lamotrigine clearance during pregnancy (From Pennell PB, Peng L, Newport DJ, Ritchie JC, Koganti A, Holley DK, Newman M, Stowe ZN. Lamotrigine in pregnancy: clearance, therapeutic drug monitoring, and seizure frequency. Neurology. 2008 May 27;70(22 Pt 2):2130–6 with permission)

Reviewer's Comments

Both Author #1 and Author #2 agree in increasing the dose of lamotrigine in this patient with known partial onset epilepsy and recurrent convulsive seizure. They agree that the seizure recurrence is likely secondary to a drop in lamotrigine levels due to pregnancy-related hormonal interactions. Author #1 advocates increasing by no more than 50 mg weekly due to risk of Stevens–Johnson syndrome. The goal target increase suggested by both authors is to maintain the original pre-pregnancy levels and to control seizure recurrence. Author #1 also suggests checking the lamotrigine levels every 2–4 weeks in the third trimester due to significant increase in clearance rate reported in the third trimester with this AED [9]. Author #2 states checking the levels once a month during the first trimester and taking individualized approach based on the fluctuations in the first trimester to determine how frequently check the levels later.

As to the patient's concern regarding the added harm to the baby with increasing the dose of lamotrigine, Author #2 addresses the question by mentioning that "it is unlikely that the increased dose of lamotrigine will increase the risk to her baby as the dose changes are needed to maintain her target drug concentration." The European epilepsy and pregnancy registry (EURAP) partially addressed the question of dose-dependent risk of malformation with AEDs. A dose of 300 mg or lower lamotrigine was associated with a risk of 2 % and higher than 300 mg dose of lamotrigine monotherapy was associated with a risk of 4.5 % [11]. They found a much more significant dose dependent increased teratogenicity risk with carbamazepine at higher than 400 mg, phenobarbital at higher than 150 mg, and valproic acid at higher than 700 mg daily dose. The Australian pregnancy registry on the other hand found the only dose dependent increased teratogenicity risk with valproic acid [12].

Finally, the authors both agree in the need of lowering the lamotrigine dose postpartum. Author #1 starts the taper 2–3 weeks after delivery over a period of 2 weeks to the first trimester level. Author #2 also mentions the need to reduce the dose to pre-partum level or slightly higher within 3 weeks of delivery. In summary, the significant pregnancy-related increase in renal clearance of lamotrigine in many patients with epilepsy necessitates increasing the dose of medication in case of significant drop in levels and/or seizure recurrence. Most clinicians do monthly trough level checks and compare the levels with pre-partum baseline. There is likely a small increased risk of teratogenicity with higher than 300 mg daily dose of lamotrigine which needs to be discussed with the patient. The dose of lamotrigine should be readjusted and reduced back to pre-partum levels within 3 weeks of delivery.

Suggested Management

1. Obtain baseline lamotrigine levels in all women of childbearing age with epilepsy taking this medication; use this as the therapeutic baseline level.
2. Use folic acid at a dose of at least 0.4 mg daily in women of childbearing age.
3. Instruct patients who are taking lamotrigine to inform you immediately if they find out they are pregnant as the decline in levels may occur early in pregnancy.
4. Consider obtaining monthly lamotrigine trough levels throughout pregnancy and more frequently if the levels are decreasing, in order to maintain the therapeutic baseline level.
5. Adjust the dose of lamotrigine if the patient has seizure recurrence or preventatively if there has been a 25 % decrease in levels compared to her baseline.
6. Consider reducing the dose of lamotrigine back to pre-partum dose within 3 weeks of delivery. This dose reduction may need to begin within days of delivery if symptoms of lamotrigine toxicity occur.

References

1. North American Antiepileptic Drug Pregnancy Registry. http://www.aedpregnancyregistry. org/. Accessed 31 Jan 2015.
2. Cunnington MC, Weil JG, Messenheimer JA, Ferber S, Yerby M, Tennis P. Final results from 18 years of the International Lamotrigine Pregnancy Registry. Neurology. 2011;76:1817–23.
3. Holmes LB, Baldwin EJ, Smith CR, et al. Increased frequency of isolated cleft palate in infants exposed to lamotrigine during pregnancy. Neurology. 2008;70:2152–8.
4. Meador KJ, Baker GA, Browning N, Clayton-Smith J, Combs-Cantrell DT, Cohen M, et al. Fetal antiepileptic drug exposure and cognitive outcomes at age 6 years (NEAD study): a prospective observational study. Lancet Neurol. 2013;12:244–52.
5. Pennell PB, Peng L, Newport DJ, Ritchie JC, Koganti A, Holley DK, et al. Lamotrigine in pregnancy: clearance, therapeutic drug monitoring, and seizure frequency. Neurology. 2008;70(22 Pt 2):2130–6.

6. Veiby G, Engelsen BA, Gilhus NE. Early childhood development and exposure to antiepileptic drugs prenatally and through breastfeeding: a prospective cohort study on children of women with epilepsy. JAMA Neurol. 2013;70:1367–74.
7. Harden CL, Pennell PB, Koppel BS, Hovinga CA, Gidal B, Meador KJ, et al. Practice parameter update: management issues for women with epilepsy—focus on pregnancy (an evidence-based review): vitamin K, folic acid, blood levels, and breastfeeding. Neurology. 2009;73(2):142–9.
8. Harden CL, Hopp J, Ting TY, Pennell PB, French JA, Hauser WA, et al. Practice parameter update: management issues for women with epilepsy—focus on pregnancy (and evidence-based review): obstetrical complications and change in seizure frequency. Neurology. 2009;73(2):126–32.
9. Polepally AR, Pennell PB, Brundage RC, Stowe ZN, Newport DJ, Viguera AC, et al. Model-based lamotrigine clearance changes during pregnancy: clinical implication. Ann Clin Transl Neurol. 2014;1(2):99–106.
10. Hernandez-Diaz S, Smith CR, Shen A, et al. Comparative safety of antiepileptic drugs during pregnancy. Neurology. 2012;78:1692–9.
11. Tomson T, Battino D, Bonizzoni E, Craig J, Lindhout D, Sabers A, et al. Dose-dependent risk of malformations with antiepileptic drugs: an analysis of data from the EURAP epilepsy and pregnancy registry. Lancet Neurol. 2011;10:609–17.
12. Vajda FJ, Graham J, Roten A, Lander CM, O'Brien TJ, Eadie M. Teratogenicity of the newer antiepileptic drugs—the Australian experience. J Clin Neurosci. 2012;19:57–9.

Chapter 16
What Is Your Advice to Pregnant Women with Epilepsy Regarding Breastfeeding?

Kimford J. Meador and Gyri Veiby

Case Scenario

A 30-year-old woman with focal epilepsy of right frontal lobe origin was managed on oxcarbazepine and lamotrigine prior and during her pregnancy. She gave birth to a baby girl at full term with no perinatal complications. The baby weighed 4 lbs 2 Oz, and there were no congenital malformations noted at the time of birth. The patient is wondering about the safety of breastfeeding her baby and potential short-term and long-term risks to her baby associated with her breastfeeding.

Author #1's Response

The many benefits of breastfeeding are widely acknowledged in the general population. However, for women with epilepsy, breastfeeding remains a controversial issue as there is a paucity of data regarding the safety of antiepileptic drug (AED) exposure via breastmilk.

K.J. Meador, M.D.
Department of Neurology & Neurological Sciences, Stanford University,
213 Quarry Road, MC 5979, Palo Alto, CA 94304, USA
e-mail: kmeador@stanford.edu

G. Veiby, M.D., Ph.D.
Department of Neurology, Haukeland University Hospital,
Jonas Lies vei 65, Bergen 5021, Norway
e-mail: gyri.veiby@hotmail.com

Commentator: C.L. Harden, M.D. (✉)
Mount Sinai Health System, Mount Sinai Beth Israel Phillips Ambulatory Care Center,
10 Union Square East, Suite 5D, New York, NY 10003, USA
e-mail: charden@chpnet.org

© Springer International Publishing Switzerland 2016   133
M. Sazgar, C.L. Harden (eds.), *Controversies in Caring for Women with Epilepsy*, DOI 10.1007/978-3-319-29170-3_16

In this particular case, a mother with epilepsy using a combination of lamotrigine and oxcarbazepine, is wondering whether it is advisable to breastfeed her baby girl. Of importance, the child has been exposed to both AEDs throughout the pregnancy, and has a birth weight of only 4 lbs 2 Oz, well below the third percentile for full-term girls (WHO growth standards).

Balanced information about the benefits and potential risks of breastfeeding should be provided to the mother. Still the final professional recommendation should not be ambiguous, but as clear as possible.

The first step is to establish the mother's initial motivation to breastfeed, and identify those specific concerns that are important for her final decision. The mother appears to be motivated to breastfeed, but is anxious whether the drugs could negatively affect the infant. A drug's degree of transfer to a nursing infant can be difficult to predict. It is important to emphasize to the mother that the child's exposure will be much lower than during pregnancy. Lamotrigine is a drug that undergoes hepatic glucuronidation, and infants have a reduced capacity to metabolize such drugs during the first months of life. Studies show that lamotrigine can reach significant serum levels in nursing infants, on average 18 % of the mother's serum levels, and a somewhat higher unbound fraction [1]. Still, clinical and scientific experience also shows that lamotrigine is usually well tolerated in breastfed infants, and side effects in neonates are rarely reported. One case-report describes serious apnea in an infant that was exposed to lamotrigine via breastmilk, but a causal relationship with the child's drug exposure was not established. Lamotrigine is often used during pregnancy due to a low teratogenic potential. Two prospective studies have recently investigated developmental effects of exposure to lamotrigine via breast-milk [2–4]. Both studies concluded that breastfed infants of mothers using lamotrigine had similar development, IQ, and weight gain as those not breastfed. There was a tendency towards better outcomes in the breastfed infants at 6 months (Fig. 16.1), 3 years, and 6 years of age [2, 3]. Thus, potential long-term risks of lamotrigine through breastmilk remain purely theoretical. Lamotrigine is regarded as compatible with breastfeeding, but breastfed infants should be observed for side effects such as drowsiness or low weight gain.

Oxcarbazepine is considered moderately safe during breastfeeding due to limited scientific data on effects during lactation. There are no studies on potential long-term effects. However, oxcarbazepine has a low penetration into breastmilk, serum concentrations in breastfed infants are low, and there are no reports on adverse side effects [5].

A particular concern in this case is the combination of oxcarbazepine and lamotrigine. Both drugs are metabolized through hepatic glucuronidation, with a slower elimination rate in infants and especially those in poor health. The combination of both drugs during breastfeeding could theoretically result in accumulation in the child. Another concern is the child's low birth weight. Use of AEDs has been associated with a moderate risk of intrauterine growth restriction, but not to such an extent that it substantiates the very low birth weight in this infant. Furthermore, any adverse effects of AEDs on fetal growth cannot automatically be assumed to apply also for postnatal growth, and especially not via breastmilk. Other causes of intrauterine growth restriction should therefore be examined. Conversely, neonates with low birth weight may in particular benefit from the positive effects of breastmilk.

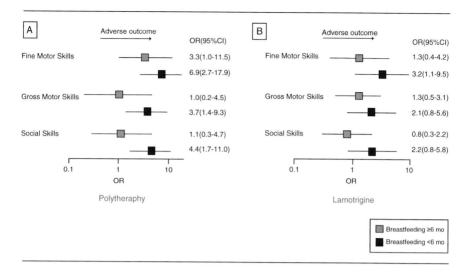

Fig. 16.1 Epilepsy groups with maternal antiepileptic drug polytherapy (**a**) and lamotrigine monotherapy (**b**) were examined. Odds ratios (ORs) with 95 % CIs were adjusted for maternal age, parity, smoking, folate use, education, anxiety/depression, and child malformation (Modified from Veiby G, Engelsen BA, Gilhus NE. Early child development and exposure to antiepileptic drugs prenatally and through breastfeeding: a prospective cohort study on children of women with epilepsy. JAMA Neurol. 2013;70(11):1367–1374 with permission)

One recent study indicates that infants of mothers using Lamotrigine or AED polytherapy benefit from breastfeeding (Fig. 16.1).

Based on existing scientific and clinical experience, the mother in this case should be encouraged to breastfeed, provided that her baby girl is carefully monitored. Serum concentrations of lamotrigine and oxcarbazepine should be measured if the infant shows signs of reduced weight gain. If side effects are suspected, formula milk supplementation should be considered.

Several measures can be undertaken to reduce the infant's degree of drug exposure. If feasible, the mother should be advised to breastfeed when drug levels are at the lowest, that is, immediately before the next drug dose. It is important to ensure postpartum dose tapering if the AED dose has been increased during pregnancy to maintain stable serum levels, which typically applies for drugs such as lamotrigine and oxcarbazepine. If there are still specific concerns about side effects, the infant's drug dose can be reduced by administering mixed nutrition, with some formula and some breastmilk.

Finally, many women with epilepsy are concerned that seizures might affect the safety of breastfeeding. Measures to avoid sleep deprivation or missed medications during the postpartum period are important. Safe breastfeeding techniques in case of seizures should be discussed, such as breastfeeding in a supine position where the child would be protected against traumatic injury.

Mothers with epilepsy are especially vulnerable during the peripartum period, and health care professionals should be careful not to exert inappropriate pressure. On the other hand, the mother should always receive information about the benefits of breastfeeding, including nutrition, protection against infectious diseases, and promotion of development and emotional attachment. Data on safety with AEDs during lactation are limited, especially for many of the newer drugs. If there are major concerns about side effects, giving formula milk or mixed nutrition can be the best solution.

In conclusion, there is no hard evidence to justify restriction of breastfeeding during AED therapy. In this particular case, the mother can and should breastfeed her baby girl, if she is motivated to do so.

Author #2's Response

The woman should be encouraged to breastfeed if she so desires. This opinion is based on the following facts. Breastfeeding clearly has benefits for both the child and mother [2, 6]. Children, who are breastfed, have reduced risk of severe lower respiratory tract infections, atopic dermatitis, asthma, acute otitis media, nonspecific gastroenteritis, obesity, type-1 and -2 diabetes, childhood leukemia, sudden infant death syndrome, and necrotizing enterocolitis. Several studies in the general population suggest that children who are breastfed also exhibit better cognitive abilities. Mothers who breastfeed also experience benefits including reduced risk for type-2 diabetes, breast cancer, ovarian cancer, and maternal postpartum depression.

In contrast, there is a theoretical concern that exposure to AEDs via breastmilk may harm the child. In immature animal brains, some AEDs can induce widespread neuronal apoptosis and synaptic dysfunction in surviving neurons [7]. These effects occur at therapeutically relevant blood levels, require only brief exposure, and are dose-dependent. Further, in utero exposure to certain AEDs has been associated with reduced cognitive abilities in children [2]. Since susceptibility of the immature brain to AED-induced apoptosis probably extends beyond birth, breastfeeding when the mother is taking an AED might theoretically be harmful to the child.

There are no animal data that directly address this issue, but studies have been conducted in humans. The NEAD study was a prospective investigation of neurodevelopmental effects of AEDs on cognitive outcomes in children of mothers with epilepsy in the USA and the UK. At age 3, it found no difference in IQ of children who are breastfed while their mothers took AED vs. those who did not [3]. Similarly, a population-based study in Norway found no effect of breastfeeding when development was assessed at age 3 [4]. In addition, the NEAD study also assessed their cohort at age 6 when cognitive outcomes are more predictive of school performance and adult abilities [2]. At age 6, there was not only no impairment, the children who had been breastfed while their mothers were taking AED had significantly higher IQ

(4 points) and higher verbal abilities (3 points) than children who were not breastfed [2]. This positive effect of breastfeeding in children of women with epilepsy is consistent with several large prospective cohort studies in the general population [2].

There are several possible reasons why fetal exposure to certain AEDs can impair cognitive abilities while AED exposure from breastfeeding does not. Since AED-induced apoptosis in the immature brain is dose-dependent, it is ultimately related to the actual drug level in the fetus or infant. Further, it is possible that adverse effects may be more related to the peak level than total AED exposure. Multiple factors affect AED levels in the child from breastfeeding, including the amount of AED excreted into breastmilk, amount of breastmilk ingested, amount of AED absorbed, and clearance of the AED by the infant. Thus, the amount of AED in the mother and in the breastmilk may not be directly related to the AED serum level in the infant. Preliminary data suggest that levels in the child from breastfeeding are low [2]. Thus, the AED levels in the womb are likely much higher than levels achieved via breastfeeding. Children whose mothers took AED during pregnancy were already exposed to their peak AED level exposure, so that breastfeeding adds no additional risk from the lower AED exposure. Further, those children who are not breastfed will not receive the benefits of breastfeeding.

Although additional studies are needed to examine all AEDs and to examine AED exposure via breastmilk for children who were not exposed in utero, the strength of present data suggests that the benefits of breastfeeding outweigh the risks. There is an unsubstantiated theoretical risk vs. known positive effects of breastfeeding, the results of the human studies showing no cognitive risks, and theoretical reasons why breastfeeding on AEDs would not offer additional risk. Based on present data, breastfeeding should be encouraged in mothers taking AEDs.

Reviewer's Comments

What can be said regarding these two Author's contributions, except that they are both internationally renowned clinical researchers who have studied the risks of breastfeeding in women with epilepsy taking AEDs and they both endorse breastfeeding for this case and in general for mothers with epilepsy. The case is complicated by low birth weight and the decision is even more carefully considered for a neonate already at risk for developmental problems. And, with caveats about what we don't yet know, what we do know about the effects of breastfeeding on these offspring, as shown by the recent reassuring NEADs data [2], leads these authors to both state that the unknown risks are outweighed by the known benefits. Author #1 discusses the low levels of lamotrigine in breastmilk with maternal use, and strategies for the timing of nursing to minimize drug exposure. Author #2 discusses the lack of translation of animal models to human outcomes regarding the effect of AED exposure on early neonatal development. This author also explains this as likely due to the overall low level of drug exposure through nursing, compared to a much more complete and robust exposure during pregnancy.

The experts have spoken and we should listen. But who is the "we?" Breastfeeding is one of the issues for which the patient may end up confused in the middle of an uneasy triangle formed by her obstetrician, neurologist, and pediatrician. Well-meaning caretakers need to get on the same page with this important issue. This requires continuing educational efforts combined with publication of ongoing research. For the individual patient, actual conversations between her health care providers are needed, so that she is not caught in the middle with no clear guidance.

Suggested Management

1. There is no hard evidence to justify restriction of breastfeeding during AED therapy.
2. Children whose mothers took AED during pregnancy were already exposed to their peak AED level exposure, so breastfeeding is unlikely to add additional risk from the lower AED exposure.
3. The mother should be advised to breastfeed when drug levels are at the lowest, that is, immediately before the next drug dose.
4. Breastfeeding should be encouraged.

References

1. Newport DJ, Pennell PB, Calamaras MR, Ritchie JC, Newman M, Knight B, et al. Lamotrigine in breast milk and nursing infants: determination of exposure. Pediatrics. 2008;122(1):e223–31.
2. Meador KJ, Baker GA, Browning N, et al. Breastfeeding in children of women taking antiepileptic drugs: cognitive outcomes at age 6 years. JAMA Pediatr. 2014;168(8):729–36.
3. Meador KJ, Baker GA, Browning N, et al. Effects of breastfeeding in children of women taking antiepileptic drugs. Neurology. 2010;75(22):1954–60.
4. Veiby G, Engelsen BA, Gilhus NE. Early child development and exposure to antiepileptic drugs prenatally and through breastfeeding: a prospective cohort study on children of women with epilepsy. JAMA Neurol. 2013;70(11):1367–74.
5. Veiby G, Bjørk MH, Engelsen BA, Gilhus NE. Epilepsy and recommendations for breastfeeding. Seizure. 2015;28:57–65.
6. Ip S, Chung M, Raman G, et al. A summary of the Agency for Healthcare Research and Quality's evidence report on breastfeeding in developed countries. Breastfeed Med. 2009;4 Suppl 1:S17–30.
7. Turski CA, Ikonomidou C. Neuropathological sequelae of developmental exposure to antiepileptic and anesthetic drugs. Front Neurol. 2012;3:120.

Part IV
Menopause

Chapter 17
Change in Seizure Pattern and Menopause

Elizabeth E. Gerard, Sheryl Haut, and Puja Patel

Case Scenario

A 46-year-old woman is starting to undergo menopause. She has a history of secondary generalized tonic-clonic seizures which started at age 14 coinciding with the onset of her menstrual periods. In the past her seizures were more intense and frequent around the time of her ovulation. Her seizures were also particularly challenging to control during her two pregnancies. She is in your office for a follow-up visit and is asking for your advice regarding what to expect to happen to her seizures in the next few years and whether her seizures will improve or worsen?

E.E. Gerard, M.D.
Department of Neurology, Feinberg School of Medicine,
675 N. St. Clair, Galter 20-100, Chicago, IL 60611, USA
e-mail: e-gerard@northwestern.edu

S. Haut, M.D.
Department of Neurology, Montefiore Medical Center, Albert Einstein College of Medicine,
111 East 210th Street, Bronx, NY 10463, USA

P. Patel, M.D.
Department of Neurology, Montefiore Medical Center, Albert Einstein College of Medicine,
211 East 210th Street, Blue Zone NW1, Room 020, Bronx, NY 10467, USA
e-mail: puj.patel@gmail.com

Commentator: M. Sazgar, M.D. (✉)
University of California, Irvine Medical Center,
101 The City Drive South, Pavilion I, Bldg. 30, Suite 123, Orange, CA 92868, USA
e-mail: msazgar@uci.edu

© Springer International Publishing Switzerland 2016   141
M. Sazgar, C.L. Harden (eds.), *Controversies in Caring for Women
with Epilepsy*, DOI 10.1007/978-3-319-29170-3_17

Author #1's Response

Whether epilepsy is affected by a woman's transition to menopause is an important and unfortunately understudied question. Menopause is defined as the cessation of all menses, dated retrospectively 12 months after a women's last menstrual period. The menopausal transition, however, also includes perimenopause, a period characterized by irregular menstrual cycles, and often involves vasomotor as well as other physical and psychological symptoms. Perimenopause includes the period leading up to and the year after the last menstrual period and can last for 4–10 years.

There are no prospective studies of women with epilepsy (WWE) as they pass through the menopausal transition. There are three cross-sectional English-language studies that examine changes in seizure frequency during perimenopause and menopause based on patient report. Two studies by Abbasi et al. [1] and McAuley et al. [2] were based on structured patient interviews. When women with preexisting epilepsy were queried about changes in seizure frequency during menopause, most reported either no change in their seizures or an increase in their seizure frequency though there was no significant difference between any of the response categories (Fig. 17.1a). However, the question posed to patients in these two studies did not distinguish between the perimenopausal and postmenopausal periods, which are physiologically different and may have unique implications for WWE. In a third cross-sectional study, Harden et al. sent postal surveys to WWE and analyzed the

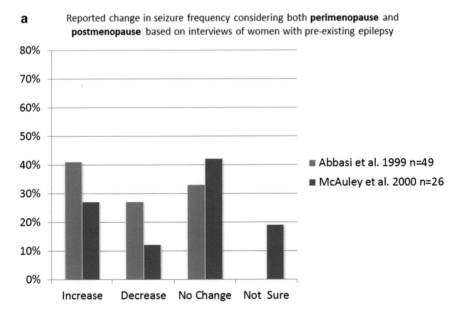

Fig. 17.1 (a) Reported change in seizure frequency considering both *perimenopause* and *postmenopause* based on interviews of women with preexisting epilepsy.

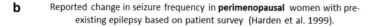

b Reported change in seizure frequency in **perimenopausal** women with pre-existing epilepsy based on patient survey (Harden et al. 1999).

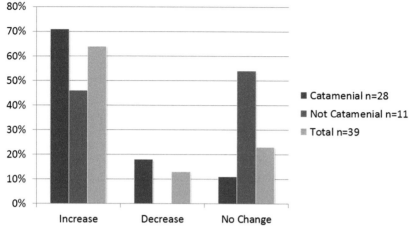

A reported catamenial pattern was associated with a reported increase in seizures during perimenopause (p=0.009). This effect persisted when patients taking hormonal treatments were excluded. Of note, the proportion of patients in this group reporting a catamenial pattern was high (72%).

c Reported change in seizure frequency in **menopausal** women with pre-existing epilepsy based on patient survey (Harden et al. 1999).

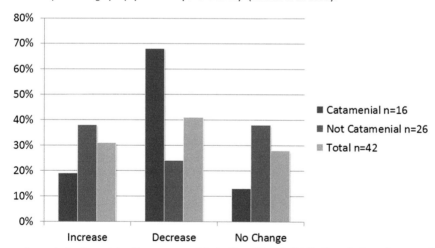

A reported catamenial pattern was associated with a different distribution of seizure frequency in menopausal patients suggestive of a decrease in seizures in these patients after completion of menopause (p=0.013)

Fig. 17.1 (continued) (**b**) Reported change in seizure frequency in *perimenopausal* women with preexisting epilepsy based on patient survey (Data from Harden CL, Pulver MC, Ravelin L, Jacobs AR. The effect of menopause and perimenopause on the course of epilepsy. Epilepsia. 1999;40(10):1402–7). (**c**) Reported change in seizure frequency in *menopausal* women with preexisting epilepsy based on patient survey (Data from Harden CL, Pulver MC, Ravelin L, Jacobs AR. The effect of menopause and perimenopause on the course of epilepsy. Epilepsia. 1999;40(10):1402–7)

reported change of seizure frequency in perimenopausal and postmenopausal patients separately (Fig. 17.1b, c) [3]. Perimenopausal WWE were most likely to report an increase in seizure frequency and the majority of postmenopausal women reported a decrease. These results, however, were mostly driven by the trends among women who also reported catamenial seizures, defined as seizures most likely to occur around ovulation, in the week before menses or 3 days after menses. A catamenial pattern was significantly associated with an increase in seizures during perimenopause. There was also a significant difference in the distribution of patient responses among catamenial and non-catamenial postmenopausal WWE suggesting that the decreased seizure frequency in menopause was mostly seen in women with catamenial patterns [3].

Despite the limitations inherent to cross-sectional studies and patient self-reporting of seizure patterns, the above studies point out some important trends relevant to this patient and other WWE approaching menopause: A sizeable subset of WWE (27–64 %) will report an increase in their seizure frequency at some point in the menopausal transition. It also seems, based on one study, that this increase is most likely to affect women with a history of catamenial seizures during perimenopause. The study also suggests that this same group may be more likely to experience a decline in seizures after menopause. This observation is in keeping with our understanding of catamenial epilepsy in which seizures seem to occur at periods of high estradiol levels and specifically elevated estradiol/progesterone ratios; Perimenopause is associated with erratic and often increased levels of estradiol as well as an increased tendency towards anovulatory cycles which are associated with lower progesterone synthesis and elevated estradiol to progesterone ratios [4]. By 2 years after the last menstrual period, both estradiol and progesterone levels reach a new and stable baseline with fewer fluctuations, which would seem favorable for women with catamenial epilepsy.

In counseling the woman in this scenario, I would advise her that based on the available literature and my clinical experience in caring for patients like her, there is a reasonable chance that she will experience an increase in seizures during perimenopause as her periods become less predictable. Her prior pattern of hormonal sensitivity may make her predisposed to this increase. However, at the same time I would explain that there are significant limitations to the clinical data available and that individual patients demonstrate variable responses to perimenopause. Furthermore, it is not clear that all types of hormonal sensitivity are the same. The predominantly ovulatory pattern noted by this patient is the least frequent pattern observed among patients with catamenial epilepsy [5] and her response to pregnancy also differs from the improvement that has been observed during this time in the majority of women with catamenial epilepsy [6]. Ultimately there is no way to be certain about her seizure pattern over the next few years. In the same regard, while I would re-assure her that seizures may decrease after menopause, I would not guarantee her this improvement. I have found that it is particularly important to explain this carefully to women with intractable epilepsy who may be surgical candidates. In some cases they prefer to "wait it out" to see if their seizures resolve with completion of menopause. This can be a risky calculation for a patient with severe intractable epilepsy given the known risks of living with seizures and the paucity of data on seizure remission or resolution after menopause.

In addition to discussing the natural history of seizures during perimenopause and menopause, it is important to discuss what can be done to maximize this woman's seizure control during the menopausal transition. This includes addressing sleep disturbance common in WWE, monitoring antiepileptic drug (AED) levels closely and avoiding hormone replacement therapy (HRT).

In a randomized placebo-controlled trial, HRT treatment with the combination of conjugated equine estrogens (CEE) and medroxyprogesterone acetate (MPA), was shown to increase seizure frequency in a dose-dependent manner [7]. Whenever possible, HRT should be avoided in WWE, which can be difficult as HRT is the most effective therapy for symptoms of menopause, especially vasomotor symptoms. Some authors have suggested that if HRT is absolutely needed, natural progesterone with an alternative estrogen such as 17-B-estradiol should be considered [8]. Low-dose birth control pills or other forms of combined hormonal contraception can also be tried, and could have the added benefit of suppressing ovulation and normalizing hormone fluctuations in this patient. Neither of these approaches has been formally studied in menopausal WWE, however.

Sleep disturbances are common in perimenopause and menopause, with vasomotor symptoms being one of the most common causes. Sleep disturbance can lead to worsening of seizure control in WWE and may contribute to reported seizure increase in some patients. Alternatives to HRT can be tried to minimize hot flashes and improve sleep. These include gabapentin and low-dose antidepressants such as SSRIs and SNRIs. Alternative explanations for sleep disturbance such as sleep apnea should also be explored and treated when appropriate.

Lastly, it is important to monitor AED levels closely in WWE during the menopausal years. Endogenous estradiol levels affect the clearance of certain AEDs such as lamotrigine, an effect that is most dramatically seen during pregnancy (and might have contributed to the worsened seizure control during this time in this patient's case). There is conflicting evidence about the change in lamotrigine clearance during menopause, with one retrospective study suggesting a decrease in clearance and others demonstrating an increase or no change [9]. Women taking any type of synthetic estrogen on the other hand are likely to have an associated drop in lamotrigine, oxcarbazepine, and possibly valproate levels and these should be monitored with appropriate dose adjustment [8].

Ultimately, until more information is available for WWE entering menopause, an honest explanation of both the available data and its limitations is the best approach. This should be coupled with an individualized treatment plan based on the patient's personal seizure history, the AEDs she is taking and the severity of her menopausal symptoms.

Author #2's Response

Introduction

Changes in seizure frequency during perimenopause remain less well studied than other hormonally related aspects of epilepsy. In this clinical scenario, a woman who has experienced seizure exacerbations related to hormonal fluctuations is now approaching menopause and wants to understand the potential impact of this time of life on her seizure frequency. The discussion will focus on the known and potential effects of perimenopause for WWE.

How Do Female Sex Hormones Affect Seizures?

The principal female sex hormones are estrogens (estradiol being the most potent estrone and estriol) and progesterone, with their secretion controlled by the hypothalamus and pituitary. Estrogen has been shown to be a proconvulsant by increasing excitatory neurotransmitters, inducing the formation of new excitatory synapses in the CA1 region of the hippocampus which involves activation of N-methyl-D-aspartate (NMDA) receptors, and altering dopamine, an inhibitory neurotransmitter [10]. Although original clinical and animal studies suggest estrogens have exclusively proconvulsant properties, there are reports that suggest it can have antiseizure effects as well, which may be related to its physiological levels [11]. Progesterone, via its metabolites, has been shown to have anticonvulsant effects by raising seizure threshold. Metabolites of progesterone regulate hippocampal neuronal excitability; allopregnanolone modulates the GABA-A receptor [10].

Is This Patient's Seizure Control Affected by Hormonal Changes?

There are three examples from this patient's reproductive life thus far which suggest a hormonal influence on her seizure control. First, seizure onset began at menarche, a time marked by the initial surge in estrogen levels. Some studies have shown a relation between epilepsy onset and menarche, in as many as 20–30 % of all female patients. Furthermore, seizure control worsened around ovulation, suggesting a periovulatory catamenial seizure pattern. Catamenial epilepsy is a term used to describe patterns of seizures which occur in association with the menstrual cycle, and has been found in about a third of WWE. In ovulatory cycles, seizure frequency has been shown to have a statistically positive correlation with the serum estradiol/progesterone ratio. Three patterns of catamenial seizures have been described (Fig. 17.2): perimenstrual (rapid withdrawal of the antiseizure effects of progesterone) and periovulatory (high estrogen

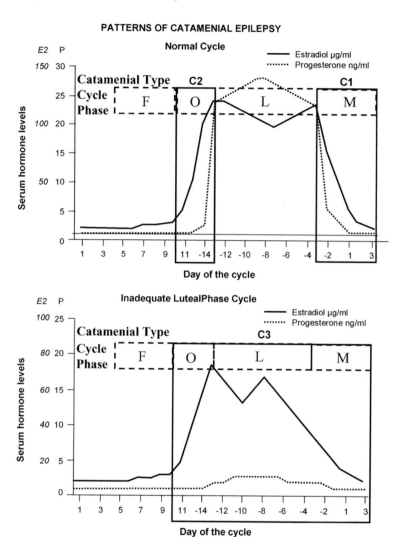

Fig. 17.2 Three patterns of catamenial epilepsy: perimenstrual (*C1*) and periovulatory (*C2*) exacerbations during normal ovulatory cycles and entire second half of the cycle (*C3*) exacerbation during inadequate luteal phase cycles where Day 1 is the first day of menstrual flow and Day 14 is the day of ovulation (From Herzog AG. Catamenial epilepsy: definition, prevalence pathophysiology and treatment. Seizure. 2008 Mar;17(2):151–9 with permission)

levels and low progesterone levels) in normal cycles, and luteal in inadequate luteal phase cycles (inadequate progesterone) [12]. Lastly, this patient's seizures were difficult to control during pregnancy, another major event in a woman's reproductive life, with 15–30 % of WWE having an increase in seizure frequency during pregnancy. Pregnancy-induced changes in AED pharmacokinetics are a major factor affecting seizure control, although compliance with or changes in AEDs for concerns of teratogenicity, or stressors during pregnancy including sleep deprivation also play a role [11]. Given this history, the concern that menopause may further affect her seizure frequency appears well founded and deserving of further thought in regard to hormonal changes during menopause.

What Hormonal Changes Occur During Menopause?

Perimenopause is characterized by menstrual irregularity and increasing anovulatory cycles during which circulating estrogen levels gradually decline. This estrogen tends to decline in an irregular manner, and is accompanied by a similar decline in cyclical luteal phase progesterone surges. The estrogen/progesterone ratio rises and generally becomes unpredictable. This process culminates in natural menopause, which is defined as no menses for 12 consecutive months without obvious cause. The postmenopausal period is marked by stable low levels of circulating estrogen [10].

What Is the Available Data on How Menopause Affects Epilepsy?

There is scant and conflicting data about the impact of menopause on epilepsy, with mostly retrospective questionnaire and interview studies which are naturally susceptible to limitations. In a questionnaire study of WWE currently in perimenopause or menopause, it was found that the majority of perimenopausal women reported an increase in seizure frequency, while in menopausal women approximately a similar number of women had no change, increase, or decrease in their seizure frequency. For women with catamenial epilepsy however, an association was found with seizure increase in perimenopause and decrease after menopause (Fig. 17.3). No revealing factors were found between subgroups of patients based on seizure type [3]. Meanwhile, other studies have not shown a change in seizure frequency or severity between perimenopausal and menopausal women, or no consistent effect of menopause on seizure frequency [13].

How Do We Explain These Results?

The increased estrogen/progesterone ratio during perimenopause may account for an increase in seizure frequency during this time. With the stable low levels of circulating estrogen during postmenopause, a decrease in seizure frequency would be expected. However, this may not occur, given data showing that the expression of

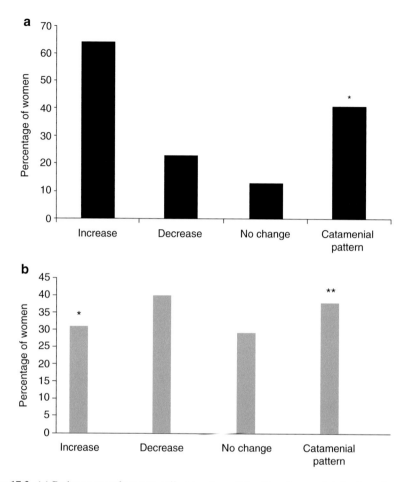

Fig. 17.3 (**a**) Perimenopausal women-epilepsy pattern. *Significantly associated with an increase in seizures ($p-0.02$). (**b**) Postmenopausal women—epilepsy pattern. **Significantly associated with a decrease in seizures ($p-0.013$). *Hormone replacement therapy (HRT) was associated with seizure exacerbation ($p-0.001$) (From Harden CL. Issues for mature women with epilepsy. Int Rev Neurobiol. 2008; 83: 385–95 with permission)

steroidogenic acute regulatory protein increases with aging in many brain regions, especially prominent in the hippocampus and cerebral cortex, areas associated with seizure initiation and propagation. This suggests active local production of sex hormones, including estradiol may contribute to an increase in seizures in some postmenopausal women. In addition, estrone is the primary estrogen after menopause with its main source being subcutaneous fat. This may be of importance for WWE who are overweight, although an altered ratio of estradiol/estriol/estrone has not been investigated [13].

Should Hormone Replacement Therapy Be Considered in This Patient?

HRT is used in elderly women with the major reason being the prevention of osteoporosis and improvement of vasomotor symptoms. Its use in WWE has been studied, showing that combined estrogen plus progesterone HRT is associated with a dose-related increase in seizure frequency [11], therefore should not be recommended in this patient.

Conclusion

The data presented is most consistent with the concept that the subset of women with catamenial epilepsy are especially sensitive to endogenous hormonal changes, correlating with increased seizures in response to hormonal fluctuations, but decreased seizures when reproductive hormones stabilize [11]. In these women, therefore, an increase in seizures at perimenopause may be expected. This effect will resolve for many of these women when they reach full menopause. Counseling with this patient should include a discussion of these factors, with reassurance that a perimenopausal increase in seizure frequency may be transient.

Reviewer's Comments

An important question posed by women with catamenial epilepsy is whether their seizures improve when they reach menopause. Both authors have addressed the importance of distinguishing perimenopausal period from menopause when counseling these patients. Author #1 mentions the lack of conclusive prospective studies on this issue. Both authors refer to the available cross-sectional studies in the literature which are mostly based on interviews and retrospective questionnaires. The study by Harden and colleagues is the only one out of the three which addressed the perimenopausal and menopausal periods separately and found that the majority of perimenopausal women reported an increase in seizure frequency, while menopausal women with catamenial epilepsy reported seizure improvement compared to their baseline.

Both authors discourage this patient from using hormonal replacement therapy. This recommendation is based on the results of randomized, double-blind, placebo-controlled trial of the effect of HRT on seizure frequency in postmenopausal WWE, taking stable doses of AEDs, and within 10 years of their last menses [7]. The study found dose dependent worsening of seizures in this population of women. In case of absolute need for hormonal therapy for vasomotor symptoms related to perimenopause, Author #1 and some other experts advocate natural progesterone with an alternative estrogen such as 17-β-estradiol [8] or low-dose birth control to suppress ovulation and prevent hormonal fluctuations. In counseling women with catamenial epilepsy who undergo perimenopause, adjusting the AED levels, and sleep hygiene are also considered essential subjects to address.

Suggested Management

1. Counsel patients with established catamenial epilepsy regarding the potential for worsening their seizures during perimenopause.
2. Check seizure medication levels and adjust if there are fluctuations compared to the patient's baseline levels.
3. Address issues regarding importance of good sleep hygiene in patients who experience sleep disturbance related to vasomotor symptoms during perimenopause. Recommend low-dose antidepressants or sleep medications if necessary.
4. Do not use hormonal replacement therapy (HRT) in perimenopausal WWE.
5. If the hot flashes are severe and disturbing, consider natural progesterone in addition to 17-β-estradiol or low-dose oral contraceptives.
6. There is some evidence that after menopause is completed and hormonal status is stabilized the seizures may improve but individual variability may exist.

Disclosures Dr. Gerard is a consultant for an investigator-initiated trial sponsored by UCB Pharma. She is also the site-PI for a trial sponsored by SAGE pharmaceuticals. She also received funding from NINDS grant U01 NS038455.

References

1. Abbasi F, Krumholz A, Kittner SJ, Langenberg P. Effects of menopause on seizures in women with epilepsy. Epilepsia. 1999;40(2):205–10.
2. McAuley JW, Koshy SJ, Moore JL, Peebles CT, Reeves AL. Characterization and health risk assessment of postmenopausal women with epilepsy. Epilepsy Behav. 2000;1(5):353–5.
3. Harden CL, Pulver MC, Ravelin L, Jacobs AR. The effect of menopause and perimenopause on the course of epilepsy. Epilepsia. 1999;40(10):1402–7.
4. Burger HG, Hale GE, Dennerstein L, Robertson DM. Cycle and hormone changes during perimenopause: the key role of ovarian function. Menopause. 2008;15(4 Pt 1):603–12.
5. Herzog AG. Catamenial epilepsy: update on prevalence, pathophysiology and treatment from the findings of the NIH Progesterone Treatment Trial. Seizure. 2015;28:18–25.
6. Cagnetti C, Lattanzi S, Foschi N, Provinciali L, Silvestrini M. Seizure course during pregnancy in catamenial epilepsy. Neurology. 2014;83(4):339–44.
7. Harden CL, Herzog AG, Nikolov BG, Koppel BS, Christos PJ, Fowler K, et al. Hormone replacement therapy in women with epilepsy: a randomized, double-blind, placebo-controlled study. Epilepsia. 2006;47(9):1447–51.
8. Harden CL. Hormone replacement therapy: will it affect seizure control and AED levels? Seizure. 2008;17(2):176–80.
9. Sveinsson O, Tomson T. Epilepsy and menopause: potential implications for pharmacotherapy. Drugs Aging. 2014;31(9):671–5.

10. Cramer JA, Gordon J, Schachter S, Devinsky O. Women with epilepsy: hormonal issues from menarche through menopause. Epilepsy Behav. 2007;11(2):160–78.
11. Gidal BE, Harden CL, editors. Epilepsy in women: the scientific basis for clinical management (Int Rev Neurobiol). San Diego: Academic Press; 2008.
12. Herzog AG. Catamenial epilepsy: definition, prevalence pathophysiology and treatment. Seizure. 2008;17(2):151–9.
13. Roste LS, Tauboll E, Svalheim S, Gjerstad L. Does menopause affect the epilepsy? Seizure. 2008;17(2):172–5.

Chapter 18
Perimenopausal Symptoms in Women with Epilepsy

Nitin K. Sethi and Mark S. Yerby

Case Scenario

A 47-year-old woman with Juvenile Myoclonic Epilepsy (JME) is treated with levetiracetam and experiencing irregular menstrual cycles and severe symptoms of intermittent hot flushes. She is prescribed estrogen replacement therapy (ERT) and topical estrogen by her gynecologist. She made an appointment with me as her epileptologist and has several questions regarding the safety of using the ERT/topical estrogen and whether her epilepsy will be exacerbated by using the prescribed hormonal therapies.

Author #1's Response

Background

Women may have changes in seizure threshold related to their menstrual cycle as well as at other times in reproductive life: puberty, pregnancy, and menopause, when there are changes in the estrogen and progesterone levels [1]. Hormones

N.K. Sethi, M.D., M.B.B.S., F.A.A.N.
Department of Neurology, New York-Presbyterian Hospital, Weill Cornell Medical Center, 525 East 68th Street, New York, NY 10065, USA
e-mail: sethinitinmd@hotmail.com

M.S. Yerby, M.D., M.P.H.
North Pacific Epilepsy Research, 63705 Deschotes Market Road, Bend, OR 97701, USA
e-mail: yerby@seizures.net

Commentator: C.L. Harden, M.D. (✉)
Mount Sinai Health System, Mount Sinai Beth Israel Phillips Ambulatory Care Center, 10 Union Square East, Suite 5D, New York, NY 10003, USA
e-mail: charden@chpnet.org

© Springer International Publishing Switzerland 2016
M. Sazgar, C.L. Harden (eds.), *Controversies in Caring for Women with Epilepsy*, DOI 10.1007/978-3-319-29170-3_18

may influence epilepsy and epilepsy may effect hormones. Estrogen can be a very potent proconvulsant, while progesterone can demonstrate anticonvulsant properties [2]. With the development of puberty gonadotropin-releasing hormone (GnRH) is secreted by the hypothalamus and stimulates the release of follicle-stimulating hormone (FSH) by the pituitary. FSH in turn stimulates formation of the ovarian follicles, which secrete estradiol as they develop. This results in a surge of luteinizing hormone (LH), which induces oocyte maturation, ovulation, and conversion of the follicle into the corpus luteum. Following ovulation, the luteal phase commences as the corpus luteum secretes progesterone. Progesterone inhibits secretion of GnRH, FSH, and LH. If there is no pregnancy, the corpus luteum regresses and production of progesterone and estradiol decline. When the progesterone secretion tapers off the cycle repeats [3]. Menopause is defined as a year of amenorrhea. Perimenopause is characterized clinically first by changes in flow and cycle length, then by irregular menses, with increasing months of missed periods, the experience of "hot flashes" or vasomotor symptoms for some women, and mood changes [4]. During the perimenopause period, circulating estrogen levels decline gradually [5]. The estrogen/progesterone ratio becomes unpredictable. As a result, there can be great variability in the effect of perimenopause on epilepsy.

There are a subset of women whose seizures are clearly effected by their menstrual cycle and are said to have catamenial epilepsy. The proportion of such patients varies widely in the literature ranging from 10 to 72 %. There are said to be three distinct patterns: in women with normal menstrual cycles some have seizures perimenstrually (days −3 to +3), others at ovulation (days 10–13); in women with inadequate luteal phase cycles, they may have exacerbations throughout the latter half (luteal phase) of the menstrual cycle. Women with catamenial epilepsy are felt to be more vulnerable to seizure exacerbation in the perimenopausal period.

Potential Effect of Estrogen on Epilepsy

Therefore most women with epilepsy find no significant change in seizure frequency during perimenopause. The use of estrogen supplements to ameliorate perimenopausal symptoms seldom effects seizure frequency. Thus unless this patient has catamenial epilepsy she has little to fear of estrogen adversely impacting her seizure control.

Potential Effects of Epilepsy on Estrogen Replacement

Epilepsy itself or seizures have little or no effect on the concentrations of estrogens either "natural" or supplemental.

Potential Effects of Antiepilepsy Medication (AED) on Estrogen

Oral contraceptives have not been associated with exacerbation of epilepsy [6]. The effectiveness of hormonal contraceptives can however, be reduced by enzyme-inducing AED (carbamazepine, phenytoin, phenobarbital, felbamate, topiramate). Hormonal contraceptives come in several formulations: oral (estrogen–progesterone combinations, or progesterone only); subcutaneous; intravaginal; intrauterine; and injectable (depoprovera). All of these forms except intravaginal and intrauterine can be adversely impacted by enzyme-inducing AED.

Enzyme-inducing AEDs may lower concentrations of estrogens by 40–50 %. They also increase sex hormone-binding globulin (SHBG) which increases the binding of progesterone and reducing the unbound fraction. The result is that hormonal contraception is less reliable with enzyme-inducing AED.

This patient is taking levetiracetam, an AED with no enzyme induction or inhibition, and thus should not affect the concentration of supplemental estrogen.

Specific Counseling and Treatment Recommendations

Assuming that this patient's epilepsy is well controlled and that she does not have catamenial epilepsy, one would not expect any exacerbation of her seizures from estrogen supplementation. Estrogen supplementation if properly dosed is safe and effective, but there is a small risk of increased rates of cancer. This risk is strongly influenced by family history and a careful history of female cancers in the family should be taken. The use of topical estrogen cream may help reduce vaginal dryness. Her other perimenopausal symptoms particularly the hot flushes maybe controlled by alternative pharmacological therapies such as gabapentin particularly extended release formulations such as Gralise or SSRIs. The irregularity of her cycles is part of the natural process of aging; many clinicians prefer to manage the symptoms with ERT or letting the natural process of menopause play out. However recent studies have demonstrated that there is a tremendous variation in the duration of perimenopause and menopausal symptoms. Ethnicity appears to have some impact on this. Thus the symptoms particularly hot flashes may last months to years and the discomfort of these should not be minimized.

Author #2's Response

Peri- and postmenopausal women at times experience distressing symptoms such as hot flashes, night sweats, vaginal dryness, urinary urgency, insomnia, weight gain, and labile mood due to decrease in the level of reproductive steroids. High turnover osteoporosis too may occur after menopause. All these factors lead to consideration of ERT and topical estrogen in these women.

Reproductive hormones estrogen and progesterone have neuroactive properties that modulate neuronal excitability affecting seizure frequency during the lifetime of a woman with epilepsy (WWE). While estradiol acts as a proconvulsant by increasing excitatory glutamate receptor activity through augmentation of N-methyl-D-aspartate receptors and inhibiting GABA synthesis through reduction of glutamic acid decarboxylase, progesterone metabolite tetrahydro-progestrone increases seizure threshold by increasing GABA-mediated chloride conductance. Thus, in peri- and postmenopausal WWE careful thought has to be given before prescribing ERT as the fear is that ERT may exacerbate seizure frequency in these women [5, 7].

JME or Janz syndrome is a common idiopathic-generalized epilepsy syndrome characterized by myoclonic jerks which are most prominent on waking up in the morning. In addition these patients suffer from generalized tonic-clonic seizures and absence seizures. While valproic acid is the most effective anticonvulsant, WWE of childbearing age are frequently treated with either lamotrigine or levetiracetam due to concern for fetal malformations with valproic use during pregnancy. Treatment is usually lifelong though recent studies indicate that in a significant minority of these patients seizure tendency may abate later in life allowing anticonvulsant therapy to be gradually weaned off over time.

A woman's baseline seizure frequency and control may change at the time of menopause. As anovulatory cycles develop, it leads to an increased estrogen to progesterone ratio theoretically increasing seizure tendency. Later in the course of menopause, estrogen production declines progressively which theoretically may lead to better seizure control and decreased seizure tendency. Women who have hormonally sensitive epilepsy with exacerbation of seizures/clustering of seizures around the menstrual cycle, a pattern known as catamenial epilepsy are more likely to experience a change in their seizure frequency during menopause [8, 9].

Our patient is a 47-year-old woman with JME on levetiracetam who is perimenopausal and experiencing severe distressing symptoms of hot flushes and vaginal dryness. She is prescribed ERT and topical estrogen by her gynecologist and is concerned it may exacerbate her underlying seizure disorder. Though not specifically indicated, I shall assume for the case of discussion that her seizures are well controlled on levetiracetam at 750 mg twice daily. Level when checked 3 months ago was 23 (range 12–46 µg/mL). Her last generalized convulsion was 5 years ago and occurred in the setting of medication noncompliance. She is tolerating levetiracetam well and denies any side effects. I shall begin by counseling her on the neuroactive properties of reproductive hormones specifically estrogen (estradiol) and what effect HRT (conjugated estrogen and medroxyprogesterone) can have on seizure frequency. If she has a catamenial pattern to her seizure disorder, she is more likely to experience an initial increase in her seizure frequency during perimenopause as anovulatory cycles cause an increase in estrogen to progesterone ratio. Administration of ERT at this time can worsen seizure control by further lowering seizure threshold [10]. I would keep her under close follow-up as ERT is commenced and if seizure control deteriorates, I would increase levetiracetam dose aiming for blood level in the high therapeutic range. Alternatively if she is very apprehensive about her seizure control deteriorating, I may consider prophylactically increasing her levetiracetam dose prior to commencement of ERT.

If she denies a catamenial pattern to her seizure disorder, I would have a discussion with her weighing the potential benefits of HRT/ERT against potential risks in the perimenopausal and postmenopausal stage (symptom control vs. seizure control). Low-dose ERT can be initiated under close observation if perimenopausal symptoms are particularly distressing. I shall prognosticate her that during perimenopausal anovulation she may experience an increase in seizure frequency if ERT leads to a further increase in estrogen/progesterone ratio. She can expect a decrease in seizure frequency during menopause as estrogen levels fall. If perimenopausal symptoms are not particularly distressing it shall be best to wait till menopause when estrogen levels fall. At that time ERT can be given safely. If perimenopausal symptoms are so distressing that ERT cannot be avoided, supplementing low-dose natural progesterone along with ERT, may ameliorate symptoms without lowering seizure threshold [11].

Reviewer's Comments

These two authors have both presented the potential neurosteroid effects of reproductive hormones on seizure occurrence at perimenopause and menopause. For women in their reproductive years, the cyclic hormonal changes that result in menstruation produce a complex, dynamic neurophysiologic milieu. Therefore impact of exogenous hormones on seizures during this hormonally tumultuous female reproductive life epoch is difficult to discern. For example, the study of natural progesterone treatment for catamenial seizures did not achieve the endpoint of proving that it is associated with seizure reduction [12]. This result is likely not because the theoretical approach is wrong, but that the study population is very heterogeneous. In fact, a follow-up post hoc report found a more defined subgroup of study subjects, who had a Type 1 catamenial seizure pattern, who responded well to natural progesterone [13].

In contrast, during the menopausal epoch, the hormonal milieu is stable. The impact of exogenous hormones in the menopausal state, with the use of conjugated equine estrogens (CEE) and medroxyprogesterone acetate (MPA) as hormone replacement, is fairly clear, in that even with very small numbers of subjects, a dose-associated increase in seizures occurred [8].

Both authors clearly presented the working hypotheses that would explain seizure change during perimenopause and menopause and put forth management strategies that are sensible, and cautious regarding mitigating seizure risk, and further, respectful of her hormone-associated difficulties at this time in her life. Both authors suggested treatments for the perimenopausal symptoms, but with CEE. Although other forms of estrogen replacement have not been well-studied in women with epilepsy, the use of estradiol with natural progesterone would likely be safer based on predicted neurosteroid effects.

Suggested Management

1. Monitor for seizure change at perimenopause.
2. Consider preventatively increasing AED dose depending on clinical scenario; a history of catamenial seizure pattern strengthens this consideration.
3. Treat perimenopausal symptoms with hormone alternatives.
4. If hormone replacement is necessary, use estradiol with natural progesterone supplementation.

Disclosures N.K. Sethi serves as Associate Editor, The Eastern Journal of Medicine

References

1. Blackstrom T. Epileptic seizures in women related to plasma estrogen and progesterone during the menstrual cycle. Acta Neurol Scand. 1976;54:321–47.
2. Logothetis J, Harner R, Morrell F, Torres F. The role of estrogens in catamenial exacerbation of epilepsy. Neurology. 1959;9:352–60.
3. Foldvary-Schaefer N, Falcone T. Catamenial epilepsy: pathophysiology, diagnosis, and management. Neurology. 2003;61(6 Suppl 2):S2–15.
4. Mitchell ES, Woods NE, Mariella A. Three stages of menopausal transition from the Seattle Midlife Women's Health Study: toward a more precise definition. Menopause. 2000;7:334–49.
5. Harden CL, Pulver MC, Ravdin L, Jacobs AR. The effect of menopause and perimenopause on the course of epilepsy. Epilepsia. 1999;40(10):1402–7.
6. Mattson RH, Cramer JA, Darney PD, Naftolin F. Use of oral contraceptives by women with epilepsy. JAMA. 1986;256(2):238–40.
7. Abbasi F, Krumholz A, Kittner SJ, Langenberg P. Effects of menopause on seizures in women with epilepsy. Epilepsia. 1999;40:205–10.
8. Harden CL, Herzog AG, Nikolov BG, Koppel BS, Christos PJ, Fowler K, Labar DR, Hauser WA. Hormone replacement therapy in women with epilepsy: a randomized, double-blind, placebo-controlled study. Epilepsia. 2006;47(9):1447–51.
9. Herzog AG. Menstrual disorders in women with epilepsy. Neurology. 2006;66(6 Suppl 3):S23–8.
10. Harden CL, Koppel BS, Herzog AG, Nikolov BG, Hauser WA. Seizure frequency is associated with age at menopause in women with epilepsy. Neurology. 2003;61:451–5.
11. Herzog AG. Reproductive endocrine considerations and hormonal therapy for women with epilepsy. Epilepsia. 1991;32 Suppl 6:S27–33.
12. Herzog AG, Fowler KM, Smithson SD, Kalayjian LA, Heck CN, Sperling MR, Liporace JD, Harden CL, Dworetzky BA, Pennell PB, Massaro JM, Progesterone Trial Study Group. Progesterone vs placebo therapy for women with epilepsy: a randomized clinical trial. Neurology. 2012;78(24):1959–66.
13. Herzog AG. Catamenial epilepsy: update on prevalence, pathophysiology and treatment from the findings of the NIH Progesterone Treatment Trial. Seizure. 2015;28:18–25.

Chapter 19
Bone Health in Women with Epilepsy

Pamela Crawford and Enrique A. Serrano

Case Scenario

A 55-year-old woman has been on carbamazepine for 30 years with excellent control of her partial-onset seizures. In the past when an attempt was made to switch her to lamotrigine or levetiracetam, she experienced seizure recurrence as soon as carbamazepine was tapered off. You order vitamin D levels which are borderline low and a DXA scan which shows osteoporosis of hip and thoracic spine. What is your advice to her for future management of her epilepsy in this context?

Author #1's Response

Antiepileptic drugs (AEDs) are associated with increased rates of bone loss and abnormalities in bone and mineral metabolism. This case presents a difficult problem in that the patient has developed osteoporosis in part secondary to her AED

P. Crawford, M.B. Ch.B., M.D., F.R.C.P.
Retired Consultant Neurologist, Department of Neurosciences,
York Hospital, Wigginton Road, York, UK, YO61 4TA
e-mail: pcrawford@doctors.org.uk

E.A. Serrano, M.D.
Department of Neurology, Comprehensive Epilepsy Center, University of Miami,
Miller School of Medicine, 1120 NW 14th Street, Clinical Research Building,
Miami, FL 33136, USA
e-mail: eserrano4@med.miami.edu

Commentator: M. Sazgar, M.D. (✉)
University of California, Irvine Medical Center,
101 The City Drive South, Pavilion I, Bldg. 30, Suite 123, Orange, CA 92868, USA
e-mail: msazgar@uci.edu

© Springer International Publishing Switzerland 2016
M. Sazgar, C.L. Harden (eds.), *Controversies in Caring for Women with Epilepsy*, DOI 10.1007/978-3-319-29170-3_19

therapy and has had two failed attempts to change her epilepsy medication to AEDs that are unlikely to affect bone density. There are two issues that need discussion. The first is the management of her epilepsy and what she would like to do next; the second is to try and optimize her bone health.

As with any new consultation, I would begin by taking a history of the seizure disorder, seizure precipitants, and AED history. It is stated that she has partial-onset seizures and I would ask if she had any warning in the form of simple partial seizures or if there were any risk factors that might make her more prone to partial-onset epilepsy. In these circumstances, intermittent clobazam therapy (5 or 10 mg) can be useful in preventing predictable seizures if further attempts at changes in AED therapy were to be undertaken.

This lady has had two failed attempts at changing her AEDs. I would look at whether this could have been achieved more successfully, for instance if she had needed a high dose of carbamazepine to initially control her seizures then it is likely she would need a dose of 400–500 mg of lamotrigine or 2000–3000 mg of levetiracetam daily to achieve the same degree of seizure freedom. Sometimes the background AED is reduced as the new AED is introduced or the reduction of the background AED can be fast precipitating withdrawal seizures. However having had two failed attempts at changing AED therapy, realistically it is unlikely that she would agree to further attempts at changing her medication unless there had been major flaws in previous management. If a further change was to be attempted, I would discuss with her the possibility that if she had further seizures then she could injure herself and there is a very small risk of sudden unexpected death in epilepsy (SUDEP). There are also the driving regulations which vary from country to country and, in the USA, from state to state.

If she was willing to try again, the alternatives are now limited. Pregabalin and gabapentin are effective in partial-onset seizures and would be worth considering although weight gain can be a common unwelcome side effect. Theoretically carbamazepine analogues such as oxcarbazepine have less hepatic microsomal enzyme induction and therefore reduced effects on vitamin D metabolism and possibly bone health but this is unproven. There is scanty literature about the recently licensed AEDs and bone health. She has been seizure free for many years and epilepsy surgery is likely to be contraindicated.

As a further change in AED therapy is unlikely, I would discuss with her the risk factors for osteoporosis (Table 19.1) and non-pharmacological methods of improving/maintaining bone health (Table 19.2). Osteoporosis is defined as a bone-mineral density (BMD) that is 2.5 or more standard deviations below the mean and characterized by low bone mass which is associated with reduced bone strength and an increased risk of fractures.

Fractures are the most important clinical manifestation of osteoporosis. The Women's Health Initiative (WHI) showed that the use of AEDs (in particular polytherapy and enzyme-inducing AEDs) were associated with a significant increased risk of fractures [1]. In this study there was also a significant association between AED usage and falls. Large case-control studies have been unable to show the

Table 19.1 Risk factors for low BMD

• Age
• Family history of osteoporosis
• BMI/weight changes
• Exercise
• Vitamin D and calcium intake
• Age at onset menopause
• Number of pregnancies
• Alcohol consumption
• Medications
• Smoking
• Other illnesses predisposing to low BMD

Table 19.2 Lifestyle measures that may decrease risk of osteoporotic fractures

• Regular weight-bearing exercises
• Smoking cessation
• Limiting alcohol intake
• Prevention of falls
• Dietary calcium intake of 1200 mg/day
• Vitamin D intake 400–800 mg/day
• Avoid other medications that may decrease bone density

increased risk associated with hepatic microsomal enzyme-inducing AEDs compared to other AEDs [2]. Other studies have highlighted the increased risk of osteoporosis that is associated with older age, being female, tonic-clonic seizures, a greater severity of epilepsy and duration of AED use [3]. No single mechanism has emerged to explain all the changes in bone in association with epilepsy and AEDs. It is thought that as carbamazepine induces hepatic microsomal enzymes it increases the destruction of vitamin D and this makes people with epilepsy who are taking carbamazepine or other hepatic microsomal enzyme-inducing drugs more prone to osteoporosis. Valproate, carbonic anhydrase inhibitors (topiramate and zonisamide), and the ketogenic diet can have effects on bone metabolism.

There are many treatments available for osteoporosis but there are very limited studies in people with epilepsy. One study showed that giving calcium and vitamin D therapy led to significant improvements in bone-mineral density in men on AEDs. The men were randomized to receive calcium and vitamin D supplementation or Risedronate plus calcium and vitamin D. There was a 70 % improvement in bone-mineral density in both groups but there was a greater increase in bone-mineral density in the lumbar spine in the Risedronate plus calcium and vitamin D group compared to those on calcium and vitamin D alone. There were also five new vertebral fractures and one non-vertebral fracture observed in the group on calcium and vitamin D alone [4].

In 2008 WHO task force introduced a fracture risk assessment tool (FRAX) [5] which estimates the 10-year probability of a hip or major osteoporotic fracture. National guidelines for treatment vary, for example in the UK, pharmacological therapy such as a bisphosphonate is cost-effective in all ages when the 10-year probability of a major osteoporotic fracture exceeds 7 %.

I would calculate this patient's FRAX score but it is likely that she will need treatment with a bisphosphonate as well as calcium and vitamin D, whether she changes her antiepileptic medication or not, as she has already been shown to have osteoporosis. Her DXA scan should be repeated after 2 years to check for response to treatment.

In conclusion, I think it is unlikely that this woman would consider further AED changes so my consultation would concentrate on discussing lifestyle changes and pharmacological therapies that may reduce the risk of subsequent osteoporotic fractures.

Author #2's Response

In light of the woman's osteoporosis, switching to another AED was considered because of the potential role of carbamazepine (CBZ) in reducing BMD. This patient was able to achieve remission on CBZ but unfortunately developed seizures when an attempt was made to switch to another AED and when CBZ was tapered off. Deciding to switch AED due to concerns for long-term side effects requires careful consideration of the risks and benefits of changing the AED. Developing recurrent seizures and other worrisome complications are risks that can occur when switching AEDs.

A study by Wang et al. examined cases that were seizure free at the time of AED switch [6]. This study showed that 21.7 % of patients switching from phenytoin and CBZ developed recurrent seizures within 6 months of changing to a new AED. It was determined that the odds of seizure recurrence were about 6.5 times higher if the AED was switched than if the existing therapy was maintained.

In addition to the development of recurrent seizures from switching AEDs, there is the possibility that the seizures may not respond to the newer AED or that the prior responsiveness to the older AED may have changed and is not able to completely control the seizures as it used to. Furthermore, the newer AED may have intolerable symptoms.

Suffering from recurrent seizures can affect psychosocial, behavioral, and cognitive functions in people with epilepsy [7, 8]. Recurrent seizures can affect the quality of life of the patients. The sudden loss of independence, inability to drive, work restrictions, and aggravation of comorbid conditions are complications encountered in patients who suffer from seizures [7, 8].

Accidents, injuries, and death may potentially occur at any one time a patient suffers from a seizure. Death from epilepsy can be attributed to status epilepticus, seizure-related deaths, sudden unexpected death, and accidents [9]. Studies have determined that the risk for SUDEP is 20 times greater in people with epilepsy than in the general population [8]. In addition, studies have shown that an increased risk of SUDEP is associated with frequent changes in dosing or seizure medications and could be a potential complication when switching AEDs [8].

Bone fractures may occur as a result of accidents and injuries during a seizure. Bone fractures can lead to pain, limited mobility, and deformities potentially causing worsening in physical and mental health that can significantly impair quality of life of the patients [10]. Fractures can occur as a result of trauma related to the seizures, especially in our scenario of a susceptible woman with an already diminished BMD. Additionally, fractures can occur as a result of falls caused by toxic effects of AEDs such as impaired balance, coordination, and vision [11]. Hence, seizures and the potential AED toxic effects can also contribute to the increased fracture risk in patients with epilepsy.

Studies have shown that taking enzyme-inducing agents (carbamazepine, phenobarbital, phenytoin, and primidone) can increase the risk of bone disease in patients with epilepsy [12]. Vitamin D is converted into inactive metabolites in the liver microsomes by the induction of the cytochrome P450 enzyme system by these medications [12]. A reduced level of the bioavailable vitamin D causes decreased absorption of calcium in the gut leading to low calcium levels and an increase in PTH [12]. PTH subsequently increases bone turnover causing loss of bone density [12]. A decrease in bone density may increase the risk of bone fractures in patients taking enzyme-inducing AEDs.

It has been suggested that patients on enzyme-inducing AEDs with low vitamin D levels and low BMD may benefit the most from vitamin D therapy [13]. However, there are no current studies to assess the optimal dose of vitamin D to be used, and there are no widely accepted guidelines for vitamin D supplementation in ambulatory patients on long-term AED treatment [13]. It is recommended that doses between 400 and 2000 IU/day for prophylaxis are used at the start of AED therapy, and 2000–4000 IU/day for treatment of osteoporosis/osteopenia [13].

This paper reviewed several significant concerns from switching CBZ in a woman with well-controlled epilepsy who has osteoporosis. Discussing the risks and the benefits of switching or continuation of AEDs should be performed with this patient. The patient can then decide on how to proceed after reviewing different options in her care. If the patient decides to continue with CBZ therapy in order to prevent complications from switching AEDs, recommendations to prevent worsening bone disease and minimizing the risks of falls and fractures should be made. Due to low levels of vitamin D, this patient can benefit from calcium and vitamin D supplementation at doses of 2000–4000 IU/day as vitamin D deficiency may potentially be a mechanism for the decrease in BMD. An endocrine evaluation is recommended in order to evaluate and treat for other secondary causes of osteoporosis and for consideration of bisphosphonate therapy. Counseling the patient on fall prevention and monitoring for symptoms of drug toxicity causing impaired vision, balance, and coordination should be performed to minimize risk of falls and fractures. Performing weight-bearing activities is highly encouraged to improve agility, balance, posture, and strength to reduce the risk of falling. It has been observed that women who perform weight-bearing activities for 30 min have a significant increase in lumbar spine of 4 % when compared to bisphosphonate therapy, which increases bone density by 2–4 % per year [11]. Hip pad protectors and walking aids are also recommended if the patient is at high risk for falls [10]. Avoidance of tobacco use, reduction of caffeine intake, and avoidance of excessive alcohol intake is advised. Three or more drinks per day increases risk of falling and may be detrimental to bone health [10]. Additionally, home safety evaluation to address environmental risk factors such as lack of assistive devices in bathroom, loose rugs, poor lighting, and obstacles in walking path may also be advised [10]. Lastly, a DXA scan should be performed in 2 years to determine efficacy of therapy. If there is evidence of progressive bone disease despite treatment and lifestyle changes, then consider changing CBZ to another AED with similar mechanism of action such as oxcarbazepine, eslicarbazepine, or lacosamide. However, there are no definite human data at this time on the effects on bone density for the newer AEDs, including gabapentin, lamotrigine, levetiracetam, oxcarbazepine, tiagabine, topiramate, and zonisamide [14]. Additionally, some animal models have shown impaired BMD with use of newer AEDs [15, 16].

Reviewer's Comments

This case highlights the importance of bone health in postmenopausal women and specifically when bone health is compromised by long-time enzyme-inducing AED use. Both authors point out the challenges involved in trying to "rock the boat" and switch anticonvulsant medication after years of seizure remission. The first author emphasizes that if considering switching to a safer AED, one needs to make certain that the adequate dose of the alternative AED is utilized and the switch is performed with initial overlap of the two medications and very gradual withdrawal of the first AED which is thought to be a culprit in contributing to this patient's osteoporosis. The second author emphasizes the risk for seizure recurrence reported by Wang et al. [6] in 21.7 % of patients switching from phenytoin and carbamazepine to a new AED within 6 months of the switch. Both authors are concerned regarding the risk of SUDEP, accidents and injuries, as well as social and psychological consequences of seizure recurrence in a patient who has been stable and seizure free and counsel the patient in these regards before further attempts to change her AED.

Although phenytoin and phenobarbital are most consistently associated with low BMD [17–19] and long-term gabapentin use is associated with bone loss in hip and spine [20–22], the findings with carbamazepine, valproic acid, and lamotrigine are mixed. In a systematic review of the literature Vestergaard reported that only 3 out of 11 carbamazepine monotherapy studies and 6 out of 11 valproic acid monotherapy studies showed a significant reduction in BMD [23]. Pack and colleagues studies the effect of AED monotherapy on bone density after 1 year of treatment in premenopausal women [19, 24]. In 23 women who were taking lamotrigine monotherapy, there were no detectable adverse effects on bone turnover or BMD. On the other hand Guo et al. examined bone mass in children treated with long-term valproate and lamotrigine and found associated short stature, low BMD, and reduced bone formation. The findings were attributed to lack of mobility rather than direct effect of the AEDs. Koo and colleagues studied 61 patients with recent onset epilepsy receiving levetiracetam monotherapy and found no decrease in bone density.

Both authors recommend vitamin D and calcium supplements, although the dose is a matter of debate. In 2011, The Endocrine Society issued clinical practice guidelines for vitamin D supplementation. Based on this guideline, the desirable serum concentration of 25(OH) D is >30 ng/mL to maximize the effect of this vitamin on calcium, bone, and muscle metabolism [25]. To consistently raise serum levels of 25(OH) D above 30 ng/mL in adults at least 1500–2000 IU/day of supplemental vitamin D might be required. There is no established guideline for recommended dose in people with osteoporosis or the ones taking enzyme-inducing AEDs. A recent randomized, double-blind, placebo-controlled clinical trial on 230 postmenopausal women under 75 years of age with vitamin D levels of 14–27 ng/mL but without osteoporosis found no beneficial effects of high-dose vitamin D (50,000 IU twice monthly) on BMD, muscle function, muscle mass, or falls despite maintaining the serum level at or above 30 ng/mL [26]. To this date, the recommended dietary allowance in healthy adults aged 51–70 in the United States put forward by the Food and nutrition Board (FNB) of the Institute of Medicine of the National Academies (formerly National Academy of Sciences) is 600 IU of vitamin D and 1200 mg of calcium (1000 mg in men).

Both authors consider endocrinology consult and addition of bisphosphonate or other pharmacologically approved treatments for osteoporosis. They will follow the patient with repeat DXA scan every 2 years. Current FDA-approved pharmacologic options for osteoporosis prevention or treatment are bisphosphonates (alendronate, ibandronate, risedronate, and zoledronic acid), calcitonin, estrogens and hormone therapy, parathyroid hormone (teriparatide), and estrogen agonist/antagonist (raloxifene).

Both authors emphasize counseling the patient regarding other important lifestyle modifications to prevent falls and fractures including hip pad protectors and walking aids if necessary, weight-bearing exercises to improve muscle tone and balance, and bone density, avoiding excessive caffeine and alcoholic beverages, and tobacco products.

In summary, in our postmenopausal patient with medically stable epilepsy on an enzyme-inducing seizure medication and osteoporosis, risks and benefits of switching anticonvulsant therapy should be discussed in detail. Lifestyle modifications to decrease risk of falls and fractures should be discussed and calcium and vitamin D supplements put in place. Consideration should be given for referral to endocrinologist for pharmacologic treatment of her osteoporosis.

Suggested Management

In women with epilepsy who are on long-term enzyme-inducing medications such as phenobarbital, phenytoin, carbamazepine, and primidone:

1. Consider calcium (at least 1200 mg per day) and vitamin D (at least 600 IU per day) supplements

2. Follow bone density every 2 years especially if postmenopausal
3. Check vitamin D levels periodically

In women with epilepsy if osteoporosis or osteopenia is diagnosed:

(a) Use higher doses of vitamin D (>600 IU per day).
(b) Counsel the patient regarding the pros and cons of switching their enzyme-inducing anticonvulsant medication. Discuss risks for potential loss of seizure control and its consequences.
(c) Consider referral to endocrinologist
(d) Consider use of FDA-approved treatment options such as bisphosphonates, calcitonin, estrogens and hormone therapy, parathyroid hormone.

References

1. Carbone LD, Johnson KC, Robbins J, et al. Antiepileptic drug use, falls, fractures, and BMD in postmenopausal women: findings from the women's health initiative (WHI). J Bone Miner Res. 2010;25:873–81.
2. Souverein PC, Webb DJ, Weil JG, et al. Use of antiepileptic drugs and risk of fractures: case-control study among patients with epilepsy. Neurology. 2006;66:1318–24.
3. Persson HB, Alberts KA, Farahmand BY, Tomson T. Risk of extremity fractures in adult outpatients with epilepsy. Epilepsia. 2002;43:768–72.
4. Lazzari AA, Dussault PM, Thakore-James M, Gagnon D, Baker E, Davis SA, Houranieh AM. Prevention of bone loss and vertebral fractures in patients with chronic epilepsy—antiepileptic drug and osteoporosis prevention trial. Epilepsia. 2013;54:1997–2004.
5. http://www.shef.ac.uk/FRAX/
6. Wang S, Mintzer S, Skidmore C, et al. Seizure recurrence and remission after switching antiepileptic drugs. Epilepsia. 2013;54(1):187–93.
7. Bazil C. Comprehensive care of the epilepsy patient—control, comorbidity and cost. Epilepsia. 2004;45 Suppl 6:3–12.
8. Institute of Medicine. Epilepsy across the spectrum: promoting health and understanding. Washington: The National Academic Press; 2012.
9. Klenerman P, Sander J, Shorvon S. Mortality in patients with epilepsy: a study of patients in long term residential care. J Neurol Neurosurg Psychiatry. 1993;56(2):149–52.
10. U.S. Department of Health and Human Services. Bone health and osteoporosis: a report of the Surgeon General. Rockville: US Department of Health and Human Services, Office of the Surgeon General; 2004.
11. Sheth R, Harden C. Screening for bone health in epilepsy. Epilepsia. 2007;48 Suppl 9:39–41.
12. Pack A. The association between antiepileptic drugs and bone disease. Epilepsy Curr. 2003;3(3):91–5.
13. Mikati MA, Dib L, Yamout B, et al. Two randomized vitamin D trials in ambulatory patients on anticonvulsants: impact on bone. Neurology. 2006;67:2005–14.
14. Gross R, Gidal B, Pack A. Antiseizure drugs and reduced bone density. Neurology. 2004;62:E24–5.
15. Fekete S, Simko J, Gradosova I, et al. The effect of levetiracetam on rat bone mass, structure and metabolism. Epilepsy Res. 2013;107(1–2):56–60.
16. Simko J, Fekete S, Gradosova I, et al. The effect of topiramate and lamotrigine on rate bone mass, structure and metabolism. J Neurol Sci. 2014;340(1–2):80–5.
17. Pack AM. Treatment of epilepsy to optimize bone health. Curr Treat Options Neurol. 2011;13:346–54.

18. Verrotti A, Coppola G, Parisi P, Mohn A, Chirelli F. Bone and calcium metabolism and antiepileptic drugs. Clin Neurol Neurosurg. 2010;112:1–10.
19. Pack AM, Morrell MJ, Randall A, McMahon DJ, Shane E. Bone health in young women with epilepsy after one year of antiepileptic drug monotherapy. Neurology. 2008;70:1586–93.
20. Vestergaard P, Rejnmark L, Mosekilde L. Anxiolytics and sedatives and risk of fractures: effects of half-life. Calcif Tissue Int. 2008;82:34–43.
21. Ensrud KE, Walczak TS, Blackwell TL, Ensrud ER, Barrett-Connor E, Orwoll ES. Antiepileptic drug use and rates of hip bone loss in older men: a prospective study. Neurology. 2008;71:723–30.
22. El-Hajj Fuleihan G, Dib L, Yamout B, Sawaya R, Mikati MA. Predictors of bone density in ambulatory patients on antiepileptic drugs. Bone. 2008;43:149–55.
23. Vestergaard P. Effects of antiepileptic drugs on bone health and growth potential in children with epilepsy. Paediatr Drugs. 2015;17:141–50.
24. Guo CY, Ronen GM, Atkinson SA. Long-term valproate and lamotrigine treatment may be a marker for reduced growth and bone mass in children with epilepsy. Epilepsia. 2001;42:1141–7.
25. Holick MF, Binkley NC, Bischoff-Ferrari HA, Gordon CM, Hanley DA, Heaney RP, et al. Evaluation, treatment, and prevention of vitamin D deficiency: an Endocrine Society clinical practice guideline. J Clin Endocrinol Metab. 2011;96:1911–30.
26. Hansen KE, Johnson RE, Chambers KR, Johnson MG, Lemon CC, Vo TN, et al. Treatment of vitamin D insufficiency in postmenopausal women: a randomized clinical trial. JAMA Intern Med. 2015;175(10):1612–21.

Index

A
Absence epilepsy, 4
Acetazolamide, 22, 24, 26, 27
Adolescence
    catamenial epilepsy, 21–27
    contraception, 29–35
    onset partial epilepsy, 11–18
    primary generalized epilepsy, 3–9
Amenorrhea, 154
American Academy of Neurology (AAN), 48
American Academy of Neurology and
    American Epilepsy Society, 42
American College of Obstetrics and
    Gynecology, 41
Anovulatory cycle, 144, 148, 156
Anticonvulsants, 91
Anti-epileptic drugs (AEDs)
    and teratogenicity, 46–47
    blood level, 50
    childbearing potential, 30
    choices, 108–110
    congenital malformations, 58
    continuation of, 46
    dosage of, 46, 135
    dose-dependent risk of, 64
    during lactation, 136
    enzyme-inducing, 90
    enzyme inhibiting, 90
    on estrogen, 155
    exposure via breastmilk, 133, 136
    on fetus, 68
    induced apoptosis, 137
    and infertility, 90
    levetiracetam and topiramate, 59, 60
    monotherapy and lower dose, 46
    neurodevelopmental effects, 136
    neonates exposed to, 109
    non-enzyme-inducing, 31
    reducing hormonal contraceptives, 31
    seizure, 56
    teratogenic effects, 56–57
    topiramate and levetiracetam, 57–60
    treatment, counselling, 60–61, 108
    use, during pregnancy, 126
Apoptosis, 137
Autism spectrum disorder (ASD), 68
Autosomal dominant nocturnal frontal lobe
    epilepsy (ADNFLE), 82, 84

B
Benzodiazepine (BZD), 69
Bisphosphonates, 162, 163, 165
BMD. *See* Bone-mineral density (BMD)
Bone fracture, 163
Bone health, 159–167
Bone-mineral density (BMD), 160, 162
Breastfeeding, 133–138

C
Calcium, 161–163, 165
Carbamazepine (CBZ), 16, 90, 160, 162–164
Catamenial epilepsy
    in adolescence, 15, 21–27
    epilepsy, 148, 154
    hormonal changes, 146, 147
    treatment algorithm, 25
Catamenial pattern, 144
Centers for Disease Control (CDC), 40

Childhood absence epilepsy, 4
Clobazam, 22, 25, 27
Cognitive development, 117–119
Cognitive outcome, 109, 110
Congenital anomalies (CA), 46
Congenital malformations, 47, 68, 70, 75,
        115, 117
Conjugated equine estrogens (CEE), 145, 157
Contraception
    in adolescence, 29–35
    pregnancy rate, 32
Corpus luteum, 154
Cortical dysplasia, 125
Counselling, prenatal, 103
CYP3A4, 33
Cytochrome P450 (CYP450), 30, 33
Cytogenetic abnormalities, 82

D
Dehydroepiandrostenedione (DHEA), 88
Depo-provera injections, 16, 30, 34
Depot medroxyprogesterone acetate (DMPA),
        26–27
DXA scan, 159, 164
Dysplasia, 29, 125

E
EEG, 4–6, 12, 22, 23, 84, 110, 121
Enzyme induction, 33
Enzyme-inducing AEDs (EIAEDs), 30, 33,
        34, 90, 155, 160, 161, 163, 165
Enzyme-inhibiting AEDs, 90
Epilepsy
    fetal malformation, 46
    folate supplementation, 40
    inheritance, 81–85
    potential effect of estrogen, 154–157
Epilepsy Monitoring Unit (EMU), 22
Epileptic seizures, 4
Estradiol, 23, 144, 145
Estrogen, 23, 88, 145, 146, 148, 149
    antiepilepsy medication, 155
    components, 33
    potential effect, 154–157
Estrogen replacement therapy (ERT), 153
Estrone, 149
Ethinyl estradiol (EE), 33
European epilepsy and pregnancy registry
        (EURAP), 130
European registry of antiepileptic drugs and
        pregnancy (EURAP), 64
Exogenous hormones, 157

F
Familial epilepsy syndrome, 83
Female sex hormones, 146
Fetal malformations (FMs), 68, 69
Fetus, 68
Focal epilepsy, 11, 14, 18, 23–26
Focal-onset epilepsy, 128
Focal-onset seizure, 127
Folate, 40, 109, 111
Folic acid
    during pregnancy, 41
    supplementation, 39–43
    supplement for pregnancy, 47
Follicle-stimulating hormone (FSH), 88, 154
Fracture risk assessment tool (FRAX), 162
Fractures, 160, 162, 163
FSH. *See* Follicular stimulating hormone
        (FSH)

G
Gabapentin, 160
Generalized tonic-clonic seizure (GTCS), 4, 5,
        108, 125, 126, 128, 141
Genetic counseling, 82
Genetic epilepsy syndrome, 68
Glucuronidation, 48, 50, 134
Gonadotropin-releasing hormone (GnRH),
        88, 154
GTCS. *See* Generalized tonic-clonic seizure
        (GTCS)

H
Hepatic glucuronidation, 134
Hepatic microsomal enzyme-inducing drugs,
        161
Hormonal changes
    during menopause, 148
    patient seizure control affect, 146
Hormonal contraceptives (HC), 30, 32
Hormone-associated seizures, 22
Hormone replacement therapy (HRT), 145,
        150
Hot flushes, 153, 155, 156
Hyperandrogenism, 6, 17, 93
Hypothalamic–pituitary–ovarian axis, 88
Hypothalamus, 88, 89, 91

I
Idiopathic epilepsy, 84
Implanted progesterone rods, 30
Infertility

AEDs and, 90
   definition, 88, 94
   neuroendocrine impact, 89
   psychosocial impact, 88
   in women with epilepsy, 88
International League against Epilepsy (ILAE),
      82
Intrauterine device (IUD)
   in adolescents, 30
   copper, 34
   current generation, 35
   implants, 32

J
Janz syndrome, 156
Juvenile myoclonic epilepsy (JME), 4, 6, 39,
      40, 63, 68, 73, 74, 115–117, 153,
      156

L
Lacosamide, 17
Lamotrigine (LTG), 5, 7, 8
   dosage, 51
   elimination, 48
   fetal malformations, 50–51
   higher doses, 47
   reduction, 48
   risk of seizure, 50
   scope of, 52
   serum level, 127
   side effects, 134
   UGT, 48
Levetiracetam, 5, 7, 8, 16, 34, 50, 57–60,
      74–78, 100, 117, 121, 122, 153, 156
Libido, 89
Low birth weight, 134, 137
Luteinizing hormone (LH), 88, 154

M
Major congenital malformations (MCMs), 40,
      42, 75, 109, 110, 115, 118, 121, 122
Malformations, 64, 66
   congenital, 68, 70, 75, 115, 117
   fetal, 68, 69
Maternal risk, 108
Medical Research Council (MRC), 41
Medroxyprogesterone acetate (MPA), 25,
      145, 157
Medroxyprogesterone injection, 30

Mendelian disorders, 82
Mendelian inheritance, 82
Menopausal transition, 142
Menopause, 142, 154
   affects epilepsy, 148
   hormonal changes, 148
   premature, 91
Menstrual cycle, 23, 25, 26
Monotherapy, 6–8, 74, 115, 118
Mortality, 108
Multifocal epilepsy, 99, 102
Myoclonias, 4, 5
Myoclonic seizures, 7, 8, 117

N
nAChR. *See* Nicotinic acetylcholine receptor
      (nAChR)
Neonates, 109
Neural tube defects, 40, 41, 43
Neurodevelopmental deficits, 76
Neurodevelopmental effects of anti-epileptic
      drug (NEAD) study group, 64, 127,
      136
Neurodevelopmental outcome, pregnancy, 109
Nexplanon®, 34
Nicotinic acetylcholine receptor (nAChR), 84
N-methyl-ᴅ-aspartate (NMDA) receptor, 146
North American AED Pregnancy Registry
      (NAAPR), 102, 111, 126
North American pregnancy registry, 64

O
Oral contraceptive pills (OCPs)
   effect of, 33
   failure rate, 32
   lamotrigine serum levels, 31
   lower dose topiramate, 31
   oxcarbazepine, 30
Osteoporosis, 159–165
Ovaries, 88, 90, 91
Ovulation, 88
Ovulatory cycles, 146
Oxcarbazepine (OXC), 16, 29–31, 33–35, 50,
      100, 134, 135

P
Parathyroid hormone, 165
PCOS. *See* Polycystic ovarian syndrome
      (PCOS)

Pedigree analysis, 82
Perimenopause, 142, 144–146, 148, 154, 156, 157
Perimenstrual pattern, 23, 25
Peripartum period, 136
Phenobarbital, 17
Phenytoin, 17
Pituitary, 88, 89
Polycystic ovarian syndrome (PCOS), 88
Polytherapy, 102
Postmenopause, 148
Postpartum
    lamotrigine dose, 125, 128, 129, 131
    period, 48
Preeclampsia, 110
Pregabalin, 160
Pregnancy
    advise against, 99–104
    AEDs use, 109
    GTCS during, 108
    neurodevelopmental outcome, 109
    registry, 50–51
    risks, 100
    risk to baby, 64
    seizures
        during, 45–52
        recurrence, 111
        and risk to mother, 65–67
Premature menopause, 91
Pre-pregnancy counselling, 76
Primary generalized epilepsy, 3–9
Progesterone, 23, 25–27, 33, 88, 144–146, 154, 156

Q
Quality of life, 162, 163

S
Seizure
    during pregnancy, 45–52
    female sex hormones, 146
    focal-onset, 127
    generalized tonic-clonic, 125, 126, 128
    medications and teratogenicity, 55–61
    neuroendocrine impact, 89
    psychosocial impact, 88
    recurrence, pregnancy, 111
    tonic-clonic, 110
Semiology, 22
Serum level, lamotrigine, 127

Severe myoclonic epilepsy of infancy (SMEI), 83
Sex hormone-binding globulin (SHBG), 155
Sleep disturbance, 145
Status epilepticus, 126
Stevens–Johnson syndrome, 7, 16–17, 127
Stigma, 88
Sudden unexpected death in epilepsy (SUDEP), 70, 108, 160, 163

T
Temporal lobe, 90
Teratogenesis, 126, 127
Teratogenic antiepileptic drug, 64
Teratogenic drugs, 46
Teratogenicity, 7, 14, 46–47, 121
Teratogenic risk, 76–77
Testosterone, 88, 90, 91
Thrombocytopenia, 6
Tonic-clonic seizures, 110
Topiramate, 5, 7, 8, 29, 31, 33, 35, 57–60, 74, 117, 121
Toxic epidermal necrolysis, 127

U
Uridine glucuronosyl transferase (UGT), 48
US Public Health Service (USPHS), 40

V
Valproate, 4, 6, 23, 26, 70, 75, 90, 122
    congenital anomalies, 46
    in pregnancy, 67–69
Valproic acid (VPA), 73–79
    vs. AED, 76–77
    conception and possible adjustment, 42
    discontinuation, 117
    dose response relationship, 64
    efficacy of, 77–78
    exposure, 40
    lowest dose of, 40
    in monotherapy, 115
    in pregnancy, 40
    risk to baby, 64
    seizure
        control, 40, 41
        and risk to mother, 65–67
    stable juvenile myoclonic epilepsy, 42
Vitamin D, 159–163

W
Women's Health Initiative (WHI), 160
Women with epilepsy (WWE)
    bone health in, 159–167
    congenital malformations, 56, 57
    early menopause, 91
    infertility, 88

    MCM, 110, 111
    perimenopausal, 144
    valproic acid, 40

Z
Zonisamide, 5–8, 74, 121